Living with Health Inequalities

This book explores how people encounter, understand, live with and respond to health risks associated with social, economic and political inequality. Complementing a traditional public health approach, the book moves beyond a focus on categories of morbidity and their structural causes. Instead, it focuses on everyday understandings and actions for people living in unequal social conditions. Making use of a variety of case studies related to physical and mental health, the authors emphasise interpersonal relationships, biographical meanings and the daily tactics of 'getting by'. These are recurrently linked to the social-structural aspects of particular times and places.

The book:

- Draws upon, applies and extends the biopsychosocial approach, which is well known to students of public health.
- Respects and gives due weight to the experience in context of people who live with health inequalities, in domestic and local settings.
- Explores notions of personal agency and the contingencies of everyday life, in order to offer a focused psychosocial complement to a public health tradition dominated by top-down reasoning.

This is an important read for all those seeking to understand the complexities of health inequalities holistically in their studies, research and practice. The book brings together thinking in the fields of public health, sociology, mental health and social policy.

Anne Rogers is Professor (Emeritus) of Medical Sociology at the University of Southampton, UK. Her research interests are in the sociological aspects of mental health and illness, self-care and management of long-term conditions, people's experiences of health care, health need and demand for care, and how patients adapt to and incorporate new technologies into their everyday life. Her most recent interests are focused on addressing how social ties and relationships operate in domestic and community settings and act as a conduit for accessing resources and support for managing wellness, social isolation and mental health.

David Pilgrim is Honorary Professor of Health and Social Policy at the University of Liverpool, UK, and Visiting Professor of Clinical Psychology at the University of Southampton, UK. He has had a long-term interdisciplinary interest in mental health policy, which draws upon psychology, history, sociology and philosophy.

Living with Health Inequalities
Upstream–Downstream Connections

Anne Rogers and David Pilgrim

Routledge
Taylor & Francis Group
LONDON AND NEW YORK

Designed cover image: © Anne Rogers

First published 2024
by Routledge
4 Park Square, Milton Park, Abingdon, Oxon OX14 4RN

and by Routledge
605 Third Avenue, New York, NY 10158

Routledge is an imprint of the Taylor & Francis Group, an informa business

British Library Cataloguing-in-Publication Data
A catalogue record for this book is available from the British Library

Library of Congress Cataloging-in-Publication Data
Names: Rogers, Anne, 1957- author. | Pilgrim, David, 1950- author.
Title: Living with health inequalities : upsteam-downsteam connections / Anne Rogers and David Pilgrim.
Description: Abingdon, Oxon ; New York, NY : Routledge, 2024. | Includes bibliographical references and index. | Summary: "This book explores how people encounter, understand, live with and respond to health risks associated with social economic and political inequality. This is an important read for all those seeking to understand the complexities of health inequalities holistically in their studies, research and practice. The book brings together thinking in the fields of public health, sociology, mental health and social policy"-- Provided by publisher.
Identifiers: LCCN 2023023818 | ISBN 9780367458362 (hbk) | ISBN 9780367458379 (pbk) | ISBN 9781003025641 (ebk)
Subjects: LCSH: Equality. | Mental health. | Public health. | Social policy.
Classification: LCC HM821 .R66 2024 | DDC 305--dc23/eng/20230724
LC record available at https://lccn.loc.gov/2023023818

ISBN: 978-0-367-45836-2 (hbk)
ISBN: 978-0-367-45837-9 (pbk)
ISBN: 978-1-003-02564-1 (ebk)

DOI: 10.4324/9781003025641

Typeset in Sabon
by Deanta Global Publishing Services, Chennai, India

Contents

Preface

Everyone becomes sick or injured and then dies. We all live in societies which, to various degrees and for a variety of reasons, are unequal. That reality has to be managed. We resist, accept and muddle through in our own way, whatever our particular social status. These forms of personal adaptation reflect a mixture of serendipity and planning, with its conscious and less conscious elements.

We are thrown into a world, which ultimately we cannot control. However, some have more power than others to defy or mitigate that material constraint on their personal agency. Ultimately, biological, interpersonal and socio-economic circumstances shape well-being, and they determine when, and how, people die. Our responses to that ineluctable and common aspect of human existence are particular to specific lives and how they are lived.

The following pages offer some examples of those particularities, by drawing on knowledge from the social sciences and public health disciplines, which address the question of how we live and die with inequality. Our aim is to illustrate the advantage of this orientation, as a middle way between the reductionist risk of individualism and voluntarism on one side, and social and economic pre-destination on the other.

With all the above in mind, we consider what we mean by 'living with inequality', with a particular focus on wellness and health. Eating, drinking, breathing, moving, thinking and feeling are fundamental aspects of all of our lives. Accordingly we consider the following:

1. The *fact* of us all living in an unequal society.
2. The *complexity* of experiences and differences between and within people, over time and place.
3. The *trends* resulting from multiple influences and the outcomes of meaning, which then create a variegated picture of living with inequalities. That includes individual differences, averages and exceptions.
4. The need to focus on our *relationships* with others, as reference points of inequality, implicating both past and present.

This social-existential approach helps to fill a gap by bringing together a disparate range of relevant literature. This will not exhaust all of the material now available to public health researchers but we use it selectively to illustrate the topics of each chapter.

Much of the public health research moves from identifying health inequalities (or unequal access to health services, which is not the same thing – see below) to social justice claims and forms of policy lobbying for reform. The need to act upon evidence of health inequalities is quite understandable, but our intention is to raise questions about the mediating processes relevant to the prospects of efforts at remediation. Those processes might account, in part at least, for why public health initiatives fail in practice.

The book makes a contribution to an emerging literature, which focuses on the psychosocial, rather than just the social and economic structural, aspects of inequality (e.g., Barber 2008; De Botton 2004; Frank 2008; Helliwell et al. 2023; Marmot 2006; Wilkinson 2005). This emergent literature is important in order to make sense of the obduracy of inequality. Many politicians, grassroots organisations and left-of-centre academics have recurrently lobbied for a reduction in inequalities. And yet, poverty itself persists in relative and absolute forms, even if by economic measures globally over time inequality has reduced, as developing countries catch up with older developed ones. That political sensitivity driving the widespread analysis of inequality, and campaigns to reduce it to acceptable levels, is only one part of the picture.

Some people find themselves in places in which there are fortuitous circumstances of flourishing. Those in the 'blue zones' we describe in Chapter 2 are born into a near optimal way of living and this may or may not reflect on their good fortune. Also, we note in the same chapter that both the rich and poor often seek to identify with living in the middle. The rich emphasise their human vulnerabilities, in common with everyone, and those in poverty might avoid the demoralisation and shame of living at the bottom of society. These subjective denials of inequality, seemingly at odds with objective measures, require describing and understanding. This is not a matter of taking a moral position about those at the top and the bottom for declaring, wrongheadedly, that there is only a middle and they are in it. It is instead about trying to make sense of those processes.

A final note at the outset is that it is beyond the scope of the book to deal with two relevant but enormous bodies of knowledge. First, we do not deal with arguments concerning the putative role of healthcare, and its availability, in impacting inequalities. There is some evidence that free good-quality primary care for all, and ready access to emergency services, improve lives and can save them. For example, without universal healthcare in the UK, free at the point of need, inequalities in health would be worse than they are already.

However iconoclasts like Ivan Illich, who doubted fundamentally the worth of modern medical services, raised a set of questions about what he called clinical, social and cultural iatrogenesis (Illich 1974). This was a gauntlet thrown down to health policy traditionalists, and the ensuing debate is still relevant for any student of healthcare. So too with important bottom-up responses of protest movements, such as the Women's Health Movement and the Psychiatric Survivors Movement. Our reading is that their impact has been important, though perhaps less than expected. Women remain disadvantaged health-wise and those with a psychiatric diagnosis are still, by and large, poor and they are still subjected to coercive state control, framed as social progress rather than a human rights violation. These variants of New Social Movements, pushing for equal citizenship, may well have remained marginal because they have been utilised mainly by patients *already* better off in cultural and financial capital.

Our view is that when people become ill, then services have a role to play in helping them as individuals. However, the health of those contacting services has *already* been shaped by social conditions. The bottom line remains that poor people live shorter and sicker lives than rich people. Healthcare often mops up the pathogenic consequences of unequal societies, at a substantial fiscal cost to the capitalist system. Accordingly, the latter can neither live with, nor without, the welfare state (Offe 1984). The concern of this book is with health inequalities in everyday life, not in the contestation about the availability and function of healthcare. It deals predominantly with wellness in upstream living, rather than the downstream consequences for pathology and service responses.

Our second concluding starting point is that we are more than aware that during the twentieth century political ideologies and experiments arose, which aimed to displace capitalism or mitigate its excesses. These emergent claims for political legitimacy emphasised the reduction of inequalities. This wider literature about political solutions to the inequalities, spawned by capitalism, is beyond the scope of this book. Historically there is evidence that Marxist-Leninist experiments in Eastern Europe and Cuba did impact positively on, for example, reductions in infant mortality and the gap in educational attainment, which is a strong precursor of health improvement. However, a high price was paid by ordinary people, in terms of state persecution, denied democracy and freedom of expression. As for the clear advantages of Scandinavian social democracy in recent decades, there too inroads into inequality reduction were made. However, this may in part have been driven by the contingency of national wealth.

These caveats and disclaimers are mentioned because they raise large and important unresolved academic and policy debates, which we do not deal with in this book. We hope though that the psychosocial matters, which are our focus, complement and inform those wider debates.

Anne Rogers and David Pilgrim
Southampton 2023

References

Barber, B.R. 2008. *Consumed: How Markets Corrupt Children, Infantilize Adults and Swallow Citizens Whole*. New York: Norton.

De Botton, A. 2004. *Status Anxiety*. London: Hamilton.

Frank, R. 2008. *Richistan: A Journey Through the American Wealth Boom and the Lives of the New Rich*. London: Penguin Random House.

Helliwell, J.F., H. Huang, M. Norton, L. Goff, and S. Wang. 2023. "World Wappiness, Trust and Social Connections in Times of Crisis." In *World Happiness Report 2023* (11th ed., Chapter 2). Sustainable Development Solutions Network.

Illich, I. 1974. *Limits to Medicine Medical Nemesis: The Expropriation of Health*. New York: Marion Boyars.

Marmot, M.G. 2006. Status Syndrome: A Challenge to Medicine. *JAMA* 295 (11): 1304–1307.

Offe, C. 1984. *Contradictions of the Welfare State*. London: Routledge.

Wilkinson, R.G. 2005. *The Impact of Inequality: How to Make Sick Societies Healthier*. London: Routledge.

1 People who need people

A relational approach to living with inequalities

Introduction

All societies contain disparities of rights, powers and wealth but they vary in type and degree. The notion of inequality is understood to flow primarily from this socio-economic context, in which opportunities and rewards are unevenly distributed across different social groups. This has social consequences for reflexive human agents, who all exist at some point on an economically determined hierarchy of inequality. An examination of its consequences for people, and for the complexities of the micro-social, involves examining the fine grain of daily life.

Such an examination has been the concern of anthropologists, social psychologists and sociologists who emphasise how societies are constituted from the bottom up. Given that the psychological is inevitably linked to the social, this brings into focus both relationships with others and the flow of inner lives. As well as real-enough socio-economic sources of inequality, we can think about their impact on both relationality and the psyche of the whole variegated range of social actors, from context to context.

Trends of inequalities shift over time and place and involve social actors making sense of them in their own particular way. People attribute meanings to experiences and, in various ways, then act upon those meanings. Meanings shape decision-making and a sense of who we are, where we came from and where we are going in life. Inner lives are linked, in a rough and ready way, with social performances, and some contexts offer more opportunities than others for them. Inner and performative aspects of our lives emerge and are modified by group belonging and social networks, as well as by fluxing social influences. Fine-grain inequalities might emerge from the existential support or defeat that is experienced in daily life, and in the various ways we belong to, or are excluded from, the lives of others.

For example, the daily psychosocial aspects of society implicate matters of autonomy, a sense of personal control, the power to pursue and access resources and the opportunities for engaging and participating in wellness in daily life. Those studying health inequalities in particular, have drawn attention to a multifactorial picture of social class, place, age, sex (now typically

DOI: 10.4324/9781003025641-1

dubbed 'gender') and race (Graham 2000). These intersections reflect both supra-personal material conditions on the one hand, and the subjectively expressed meanings in biographical accounts on the other. These two aspects of intersectionality are returned to at the start of Chapter 8. This complex web, of causes and meanings, creates a variegated picture of living with inequalities and a focus on our relationships with others.

A clarification about what we are attempting in this book comes from a longstanding expert on global inequality, Goren Therborn. He makes a distinction between shared *vital inequalities* (in relation to, for example, income, clean water, sanitation, shelter and a steady food supply) and particular *existential inequalities* (of respect, recognition and acceptance or rejection from others) (Therborn 2013). The case studies offered in the following pages focus mainly on the second group of inequalities, but always with reference to the first, which dynamically shapes who we are in a hierarchy, what sense we make of it and our reflections and decisions, as we pass from birth to death.

With these starting points in mind for the book, this chapter continues by looking first at conceptual matters about living in an unequal society before proceeding with some illustrative empirical literature from public health research.

Conceptual clarifications

A starting point is that of social orders being moral orders, which is also where we end the chapter for emphasis. That is, the fact of social inequality quickly encourages blame (of the rich and powerful) or the reverse (the lack of good sense of those marginalised and powerless). However, the interest here is in describing the cultural trends linked to these common moralisations. For example, poorer people from economic necessity are constrained more than richer people about their choices. They have fewer opportunities to shift their habits in a more healthy direction. So what are those opportunity structures and what cultural norms have emerged between classes in relation to health-related conduct?

Living on the margins with little room for negotiation and fewer financial and cognitive resources, individuals tend to make decisions in certain ways for particular reasons. These situated rationalities are relevant. For example, unlike the privileged and socially advantaged, people with few resources tend to act with a sense of immediacy and even urgency, commensurate with the necessities of food, accommodation and work (Hankivsky 2007). Living close to economic necessity reduces the ability to invest in future health, whereas those who live in more affluent socio-economic circumstances and social groups have a greater latitude to think and act more strategically in building health practices (Savage et al. 2013). They are the first to have knowledge of new health risks and they have more resources to adopt new health strategies and practices.

On the notion of 'living with' inequalities

'Living with' refers to a sense of experiential continuity or persistence. The individual component of this is a sense of who we are. The relational component extends to past and present norms and expectations developed in families and neighbourhoods. These can be described as 'lifeworlds'. People tend to abide by their expectations (or might resist them), but their character varies from one group to another and from one culture to another and within them. This implies complexity of individuals and their social contexts over time.

Lifeworlds have been a focus of interest to many social and political scientists including Schutz, Elias and Habermas. For the latter, the 'lifeworld' (*Lebenswelt*) refers to the space within a person's scope dedicated to the undertaking of daily routines and social engagement with significant others. These extend to the community, the nation and wider global society. The lifeworld constitutes a domain of regulation, in which private and domestic life can be shaped by rules imposed by a context today of the escalating power of bureaucracy, corporate capitalism and mass consumerism. If this notion of *Lebenswelt* has been a useful resource to guide the task of this book, then so is that of *habitus*. The latter was first discussed by Aristotle to mean personal disposition. It was then picked up and elaborated in modern sociology by Mauss, Elias and Bourdieu who describes it as being constituted by:

> systems of durable, transposable dispositions, structured structures predisposed to function as structuring structures, that is, as principles which generate and organize practices and representations that can be objectively adapted to their outcomes without presupposing a conscious aiming at ends or an express mastery of the operations necessary in order to attain them.

Habitus refers to personal dispositions that may or may not be conscious and they are always intertwined with social structure. When we come to use this framing about people living their lives and apply it to the topic of this book, there is a range of implications, which the coming chapters will explore. A point to make at the outset is that the tendencies of habitus within lifeworlds highlight extremes of experience (of the absolute poor and the super-rich) and the tendency of *both* of these poles and those in between to normalise their humanity. It is striking how people, whatever their background, tend to emphasise ordinariness, their likeness to others and their vulnerability and angst about life. It also goes largely unnoticed. Routine social life proceeds from pragmatic necessity, without necessarily the reflection or interest of social actors. We elaborate on this point in Chapter 2.

As Anton Chekhov noted: 'most people live their real, most interesting life under the cover of secrecy'. The motivations and dispositions of ordinary people typically remain hidden from public view. We show how this is expressed at opposite ends of the divide and how they converge throughout this book. We draw on the synthesis of qualitative research to explore the micro-processes of social life applied to health across different contexts. This focuses on the expression and meanings negotiated by people during their everyday lives.

Our analysis of 'living with' draws on aspects of embodiment, food production and consumption, feelings, connections and conformity in groups or personal communities, entailing describable social practices and particular personal cognitive schemas and behavioural habits. Looking across time and space, these provide a means of understanding and explaining human action in relation to health and well-being in the context of social, economic and structural constraints.

Social networks (or 'ties')

Exploring living with inequalities requires an understanding of the location of others and the nature of the ties that bind people together. Social networks constitute a set of individuals (social network members) connected to one another, which act as the link between social structure and personal agency. Social relationships act as a supply line of resources and assistance (information, emotional or practical help) that impact on daily living including the stresses of living (e.g., illness, life events, life transitions).

Starting with the elephant in the room of economic inequalities, poverty is a barrier to the potent reciprocal exchange of resources in networks. An impact of stigma and the prejudices that surround poverty is self-exclusion, which leads to reduced social mixing and the potential benefits that accrue from having the assets of social ties. Differing ties hold different properties of support. People living in urban poverty may rely on strong kinship ties to survive destitution, in the absence of more wide-ranging sources of support. They may also form multiple weak ties, such as those between relative strangers, or people encountered only episodically. These have been found to help those in the most dire of circumstances.

For example, an ethnography conducted in the United States illuminated how evicted families frequently turn to new acquaintances for help. These 'disposable' ties facilitated the flow of various resources. However these bonds were typically fragile and transitory. The tactic of making, exploiting and relinquishing disposable ties allowed families caught in fraught situations to cope from day to day. However, it also prompted personal instability which raised misgivings amongst peers (Desmond 2012).

Whilst this and other studies show that the social networks of those experiencing poverty have access to some financial, material and emotional support, it is vastly insufficient to overcome socio-economic inequalities. The social networks of disadvantaged people offer less 'bridging' social capital to networks of influence than the advantaged (in gaining employment, for example). When social mixing does occur, diversifying networks through social context is more limited compared to those with higher incomes who have wider networks enabled by type of education, employment and greater mobility. Collective action and efficacy are more difficult in those living in poor areas in reducing reciprocal trust and ultimately reducing support (Uphof et al. 2013)

Social networks are a conduit for resources and for establishing relationships, which shape our health and well-being. They are the setting for the deployment of resources for advantageous strategic actions, the gaining of useful information, emotional support and motivational engagement in healthy practices. Networks vary then in their richness, in its widest sense, but they are certainly inflected by a person's class position.

For example, mental health is shaped in part by a person's social standing and the networking potential this implies. An example of this, historically, is the study of psychotherapy access in the United States. It showed how middle-class connections – 'from whom one knows' – enabled people to access help (Kadushin 1966). The power to influence rested with the characteristics of members of a group. This included knowing others in therapy, those experiencing similar problems, disclosing a problem and searching for a solution and sharing cultural 'sophistication' (going to plays, concerts, museums). That shared sense of being with 'people like us', gave a person with an emergent mental health problem both the knowledge and confidence in their help-seeking. In a context of fee-paying, the cash nexus was important as a condition of help-seeking, but these other non-pecuniary aspects were also very important.

A contrasting picture of network influence is evident in the help-seeking of the less well-off. The structural and personal constraints and opportunities encountered by those living in poorer circumstances are located in network memberships with fewer resources. For example, in a study of poor Puerto Ricans, solutions to mental health problems were sought from tight family structures. Services were used as a last resort in the absence of lay alternatives. Such services of last resort were more likely to be coercive and stigmatised and so are viewed warily (Vera et al. 1998). This contrasts starkly with the example discussed above in which psychotherapy was considered a valued and high-status cultural practice.

The properties of ties are relevant too. 'Weak' ties, compared to strong and intimate bonds, tend to be brief interactions with acquaintances and relative strangers, entailing lower levels of commitment and trust. However, these weaker ties might be more durable and less liable to loss over time than stronger ties. Their multiple, repeated but transient and diffuse character creates a web of support from those like neighbours, work colleagues, shop keepers and taxi-drivers. Weak ties are useful when help from a stronger tie (such as a close blood relative) is unavailable, inconvenient, impractical or unwanted. Many people manage well with mainly weak ties. For example, those struggling to cook for themselves may develop multiple weak ties in cafes and food outlets.

An example of this sort is given here from a study undertaken in an area of deprivation in the North West of England of managing with a long-term health condition (Rogers et al. 2014). An account from someone who had difficulty seeing to cook, but who had daily routinised contact with a range of food outlets, is compared favourably with the unreliability of official caring agencies and the benevolence of strong ties. This respondent was a 78-year-old male with diabetes and coronary heart disease:

> That's how I go on, like today, I go down into H, I usually catch the five to seven bus in the morning and I go into the Mall and there's three young ladies there. She cooks me my breakfast, my breakfast consists of a bacon muffin with raw onion on and a couple of cheese slices, which I put on myself ... Every day I go down there seven days a week. I don't get my breakfast there on a Sunday, I go into Wetherspoons on a Sunday and get a breakfast there. Oh, I've got friends all the way around there that I can talk to and everything.

The same respondent illustrates the 'strength of weak ties' in this part of the interview:

> I've managed to get out even in the deep snow because of the taxi companies, I know who will send a cab for me and I pay a taxi fare to go down and I'm out maybe for an hour, I might have a drink in H and then I'm back within an hour. And that's all I ever got. I got more help from the taxi companies [than social services] in the deep snow, they used to hold my arm and carry me ... Got me across it to make sure I didn't fall and the same going out to make sure I didn't fall whilst going out ... I get more help from people like that and I've got more enjoyment out them that what I have from anybody else.

This example not only illustrates why weak ties are important, it also illuminates how they allow people to retain a sense of autonomy by not admitting the focused need for a strong tie of a carer (paid or from within the family). The person is being supported but is using their agency to engage with a range of people to achieve this aim. This maintains self-respect and avoids a declaration of dependency.

One by one, those supporting the person offer small acts of polite kindness or paid service that do not require the recipient to experience social defeat. The interaction passes by virtually unnoticed, as part of everyday life for all parties. The recipient of the support in particular emphasises that they do not require 'too much' assistance in order to live with their condition. The neighbour getting a newspaper, or doing a small errand of shopping, allows life to be kept on track. When there is a paid nexus (say using a taxi), the supported person is involved in a reciprocal not an asymmetrical relationship. All of this means the sense of an autonomous self, functioning much the same as in the past, which can be retained by the person.

Forms of capital, habitus and field

Networks are not only important (in quantity and quality) but they are also afforded in the latter regard by forms of capital. Traditionally or in everyday life the term is often thought of in purely economic terms (as in 'capitalism' or 'capital to buy a house'). However, Bourdieu (1986) pointed out that the term has other real dimensions and these are summarised in Box 1.1.

Box 1.1 Forms of capital

- *Economic capital*: The material means required to undertake health-risk mitigation and manage health (e.g., the ability to purchase Apps for exercise, special diets etc.). Those with high wealth can secure comfortable housing in an affluent area free of toxins and pollution, with good transport links and easy access to good-quality health services.
- *Cultural capital*: This represents a stock of styles, skills for interacting with others and includes the attitudes and behaviours relevant to adopt health practices and the (re) production of health (Shim 2010). These are held unequally. For example, *health literacy* – the cognitive and critical analytical skills needed to process and utilise information in a health context – has been identified as deficient in those from more marginalised communities. Health literacy interventions are an attempt at increasing cultural health capital – attaining knowledge about understanding and navigating health and medical matters. By contrast 'healthism' refers to the phenomena of 'high' health awareness, expectations, aggressive information-seeking, self-reflection, a sceptical watchful attitude to traditional medicine and embracing of healthy 'alternative' lifestyle choices. This is associated with an abundance of cultural health capital aligned with assertive middle-class norms and values (Greenhalgh and Wessley 2004).
- *Social capital*: This refers to accessible resources held by members of a personal network that a person can mobilise, draw on and benefit from in their purposive health actions (as with social networks described above) (Bourdieu 1986, 2). Those with higher social capital levels can use them more strategically. High levels of capital allow for more selective, informed, internalised, long-term and strategic decisions about health (e.g., in terms of help-seeking). Individuals with higher levels of social capital in terms of social participation and networks engage in 'healthier' behaviours (e.g., physical activity and report feeling healthier physically and psychologically) (Nieminen et al. 2013).
- *Corporeal capital*: The body is a form of physical capital, an axis of inequality, a bearer of value and a socially shaped generator of division as between social groups. Bodily capital interacts with

other forms of health capital and work. There is, for example, an identified association between social disparities and unfavourable health outcomes implicating inflammatory biomarkers, infection and indicators of physical functioning and mortality (Vineis et al. 2020). Other examples include women's use of embodied strategies to avoid being the targets of fatness-related prejudice and to manage their bodies in the workplace – situations where bodies can influence implicitly being employed and promotion (Toothman 2016). Strategically managing one's body (size, shape and weight) is relevant to within-group inequalities. For example, a study of gay men illuminated the way in which big muscular or fat bodies might be celebrated in 'bear' culture, rather than being devalued in the broader gay community (Hennen 2005).

From Box 1.1 we can see that capitals take different forms and they are distributed unevenly. The better-off begin with an advantage for both financial reasons (they can buy their way out of challenges more readily) but the rich then get richer if they also have more cultural capital (what they know) which in turn is amplified by who they know. Those connections are richer in richer networks than poorer ones. Corporeal capital comes with being young fit and better off and is jeopardised by ageing and becoming ill and poorer.

As well as these co-existing and interacting forms of capital to consider, another concept from Bourdieu is relevant: habitus. This is the outcome of our socialisation and is manifest in our personal habits (hence the name) but also our ways of thinking, tastes, confidence and aspirations. These might culminate in what then becomes known as a 'lifestyle'. The term then refers both to our behavioural dispositions and to our interiority.

Applying these points about forms of capital and habitus, they are manifest in the various ways in which people manage their lives and interact with others. When people have health problems, that particular confluence of past socialisation and current ways of acting becomes evident. Its expression is context constrained (Bourdieu, like Sartre before him, used the term 'field' to indicate that situated actions occur in particular settings). These general conceptual resources are spelt out in later chapters, especially when we consider loneliness in Chapter 6.

Lay knowledge and practice

Habitus, field and forms of capital imply that lay accounts of reality and the reported daily experience of people in different settings are all part of understanding society 'from the bottom up'. When applied to questions of health and illness, the term 'lay epidemiology' is invoked to refer to the manner in which health risks are understood and interpreted by ordinary people (Frankel et al. 1991).

Lay knowledge, predicated on the recent common notion of 'lived experience', in part has been a challenging response to disillusionment and a growing scepticism about the disinterestedness of science and the role of professional authority in daily life. New social movements have drawn on this lay expertise to overturn or modify old and traditional biomedical ways of doing things in the areas of mental health, reproductive rights, the management of long-term conditions and medicine taking (Britten and Mcquire 2015; Brown et al. 2004; Rogers and Pilgrim 1991).

Lay views of social class are also relevant, as this refers to inequality of wealth and status. This importance was recognised by the Marxist-humanist historian E.P. Thompson, who noted that 'I do not see class as a "structure", nor even as a "category", but as something that in fact happens (and can be shown to have happened) in human relationships" (Thompson 1968, 9). What Thompson is drawing attention to here is that inequality is manifest in human praxis. Within the latter, people experience, report and reflect upon their own context of inequality; at least they have that potential capability and may deploy it to various degrees in their daily lives.

Thus two concepts relevant to the aims of this book are lay knowledge and lay epidemiology and there is a third. This is about an enlarged concept of 'work'. Just as capital includes, but is not only about, money, so too with the notion of 'lay work'. What counts as 'work' shapes how we think about expertise and relevant social actors (Star and Strauss 1999). Lay or 'informal' health work, is less visible and valued than professionally paid, more highly esteemed health work. Health work is predominantly seen as the purview of health professionals. This is for understandable reasons, given that healthcare practitioners are trained extensively and are socialised to acquire competence and confidence in the assessment and amelioration of health problems. That is what they are paid to do. However, it is empirically inaccurate to conflate health work with this professional activity alone. Laypeople, prior to and concurrent with professional interventions, do health work in a range of ways.

People have tacit knowledge about how to understand and deal with their health. Moreover, when and if a health condition is formally recognised, following healthcare service contact, much of the supportive and remedial work is actually done by laypeople. They include patients themselves and the networks surrounding them, including but not only their relatives. It is mundane and often may not be recognised for what it is. At some points it may become manifest, if it is at odds with professional authority about managing illness. Potentially lay knowledge and professional knowledge may come into conflict. Lay expertise might threaten the assumed singular authority of professional work (Reidy et al. 2018). Note this in relation to the adoption of insulin pump technology by young people with diabetes who may come to know more than their treating professionals.

As we noted above about the role of networks in the self-management of long-term conditions, professional expertise may be largely irrelevant to what keeps people 'on track' in their daily lives. 'Articulation work' refers to emotional work (caring about as well as caring for people) and practical support (basic 'tending' that requires no professional expertise but is learned by most of us). An implication of this in the lay arena of social action is that task-based work is more frequently undertaken by laypeople, and identified patients may consider it to be of more utility and value than that provided by professional health workers (Rogers et al. 2016).

Living with inequalities as a fact of life

Living with inequalities is about how life actually is, rather than how we might want it to be. There is an incorrigible quality to inequality. People are both aware of its negative impacts but also of the seeming impossibility of anything ever changing for the better. Even when interventions are supported in principle, little change may be observed in practice. Shifts in the inequality equation gap through state commitments to socially inclusive economic growth, have tended to be short lived and for the most part are incrementally reversed or undone (Evans 2018).

As far as health policy is concerned, genuine structural solutions are often displaced by a focus on individualised behavioural remedies. This predominant focus obfuscates the social and economic production and shaping of health inequalities. As a personal trouble the matter of inequality produced by intransigent socio-economic circumstance can be cast aside easily. Moral exhortations and lifestyle advice to encourage better health, or nip disease in the bud via individual behavioural strategies, have displaced a need for political action to deal with structural inequalities.

Indeed health movements pushing for change have arguably made only modest gains for the most marginalised groups. Community mobilisation too is frequently unsuccessful in realising sustained wide-ranging improvements, to changing health status amongst socially precarious marginalised people. They lack personal recognition and live in adverse circumstances (Cornish, and Ghosh 2007).

A sense of fatalism, relating to financial wealth, resonates as well in lay views of health inequalities. There is little doubt from participants' accounts across a number of studies of the validity and awareness of underlying reasons for the latter (a point we explore further in Chapter 2). Those reasons are structural and relate to the material conditions of the lives of ordinary people in work and in neighbourhoods. Unemployment, stressful employment, inadequate housing, air pollution etc. are all evident underlying factors known to those people most at risk of their impact. They are also well known to those who have the cognitive and economic means to avoid or mitigate these risks to health.

This lay reaction to living with inequality confirms what we know from professional epidemiological evidence. For the poorest in society, this translates into negative emotions of fear, stress, social defeat, social isolation and feelings of being judged. Fatalism and a low sense of personal control then follow (Marmot 2017; Garthwaite and Bambra 2017).

The disgusting and the virtuous

This final section deals with another recurring psychosocial matter: the moral and moralistic discourse surrounding health. This can be thought of in a number of ways. Bourdieu in his discussion of 'distinction' makes the point that we are under greatest threat from those nearby. We define ourselves against that which is close but offensive. The 'respectable' working class are threatened by the 'rough' people, who are unemployed, unemployable and sporadically criminal (what Marx called the 'lumpenproletariat') (Hanley 2017). The middle classes, with the resources, will physically remove themselves from an undesirable lower order in their housing choice.

These cognitive divisions, when acted out can create distance between people, which are framed in a different way in the psychoanalytical tradition. The notion of 'splitting' of good from bad or vice and virtue is a way of explaining how people avoid or reduce anxiety to establish and maintain ontological security (Rubens 1996). But with this comes uncertainty, when those viewed negatively enter our lives for whatever reason.

These cognitions and actions bring with them feelings of disgust about those 'lacking virtue'. An implication of this is the growth of prejudice (by stereotyping all those in the outgroup), establishing a hierarchy of trust, creating boundaries between those who are trusted and liked and those who are not. At times this extends to disgust about bodies (Lieberman et al. 2012). This distaste for unhealthy dispositions of those at the bottom of society is crystallised here in this journalistic account from James Delingpole in *The Times* (13 April 2006, 25):

> aggressive all-female gangs of embittered, hormonal, drunken teenagers; gym slip mums who choose to get pregnant as a career option; pasty-faced, lard-gutted slappers who'll drop their knickers in the blink of an eye [...] these people do exist and are every bit as ripe and just a target for social satire as were, say, the raddled working-class drunks sent up by Hogarth in Gin Lane.

Set against that disgust with a stereotyped underclass, we find virtue in the stereotyped middle class, with lythe bodies uncontaminated by nicotine smoke, exercise regimes and healthy diets. This is the opposite side of the same coin of 'distinction' or 'splitting'. Health professionals might idealise virtuous lay self-managers and deride the failings of others. From narratives about exercise and diet, to those about alcohol consumption and smoking, the moralistic discourse of middle-class professionals about poor or transgressive patients is evident. More on this point about health moralisation in the chapters to come.

Conclusion

This first chapter has outlined the main themes for those to come and introduced concepts we use throughout the book. Whilst we refer to the structural aspects of inequalities as a context or field for the lives of people, how they then live with that reality has to be accessed via their accounts and observations about everyday life. The personal accounts include perceptions of self and others, as well as being sources of understanding for those interested in public health. The relevance of the structural aspects of society can only make sense if it is evidenced by psychosocial reality on the ground and vice versa. This requires both/and rather than either/or ways of thinking about the headline topic of this book.

What is clear is that when we talk of 'living with inequalities' that immediately implicates health and well-being. Living in an unequal society is relevant both to the emergence of health inequalities and to the amplification of inequality that such ill-health and disability might then create. This complexity is addressed in the following chapters.

References

Bourdieu, P. 1986. "The Forms of Capital." In *Handbook of Theory and Research for the Sociology of Education*, edited by J.G. Richardson, 241–258. New York: Greenwood Press.

Britten, N., and K. Maguire. 2015. "Lay Knowledge, Social Movements and the Use of Medicines: Personal Reflections." *Health* 20: 77–93.

Brown, P., S. Zavestoski, S. McCormick, B. Mayer, R. Morello-Frosch, and R. Gasior Altman. 2004. "Embodied Health Movements: New Approaches to Social Movements in Health." *Sociology of Health & Illness* 26 (1): 50–80.

Cornish, F., and R. Ghosh. 2007. "The Necessary Contradictions of 'Community-Led' Health Promotion." *Social Science & Medicine* 64 (2): 496–507.

Desmond, M. 2012. "Disposable Ties and the Urban Poor." *American Journal of Sociology* 117 (5): 1295–1335.

Duchess Podcas. 2021. https://www.duchessthepodcast.com/episode/lady-emma-ingilby-of-ripley-castle.

Evans, A. 2018 "Politicising Inequality: The Power of Ideas." *World Development* 110: 360–372.

Frankel, S., C. Davison, and G.D. Smith. 1991. "Lay Epidemiology and the Rationality of Responses to Health Education." *British Journal of General Practice* 41 (351): 428–430.

Friedman, S., D. O'Brien, and I. McDonald. 2021. "Deflecting Privilege: Class Identity and the Intergenerational Self." *Sociology* 64 (1): 129–147.

Greenhalgh, T., and S. Wessely. 2004. "'Health for Me': A Sociocultural Analysis of Healthism in the Middle Classes." *British Medical Bulletin* 69 (1): 197–213.

Graham, H. 2000. *Understanding Health Inequalities*, 227. Buckingham: Open University Press.

Hankivsky, O. 2007. "Gender Based Analysis and Health Policy: The Need Rethink Outdated Strategies." In *Women's Health in Canada: Critical Theory, Policy and Practice*, edited by M. Morrow, O. Hankivsky, and C. Varcoe, 143–168. Toronto: University of Toronto Press.

Hanley, L. 2017. *Respectable: Crossing the Class Divide*. London: Penguin Books.

Hennen, P. 2005. "Bear Bodies, Bear Masculinity: Recuperation, Resistance, or Retreat?" *Gender and Society* 19 (1): 25–43.

Kadushin, C. 1966. "The Friends and Supporters of Psychotherapy: On Social Circles in Urban Life." *American Sociological Review* 31 (6): 786–802.

Lieberman, D.L., J.M. Tybur, and J.D. Latner. 2012. "Disgust Sensitivity, Obesity Stigma, and Gender: Contamination Psychology Predicts Weight Bias for Women, Not Men." *Obesity* 20 (9): 1803–1814.

Macdonald, W., A. Rogers, T. Blakeman, and P. Bower. 2008. "Practice Nurses and the Facilitation of Self-Management in Primary Care." *Journal of Advanced Nursing* 62 (2): 191–199.

Marmot, M. 2017. "The Health Gap: The Challenge of an Unequal World: The Argument." *International Journal of Epidemiology* 46 (4): 1312–1318.

Nieminen, T., R. Prättälä, T. Martelin et al. 2013. "Social Capital, Health Behaviours and Health: A Population-Based Associational Study." *BMC Public Health* 13: 613.

Reidy, C., M. Bracher, C. Foster, I. Vassilev, and A. Rogers. 2018. "The Process of Incorporating Insulin Pumps Into the Everyday Lives of People with Type 1 Diabetes: A Critical Interpretive Synthesis." *Health Expectations* 21 (4): 714–729. doi: 10.1111/hex.12666.

Rogers, A., and D. Pilgrim. 1991. "'Pulling Down Churches': Accounting for the British Mental Health Users' Movement." *Sociology of Health and Illness* 13: 129–148.

Rogers, A., H. Brooks, I. Vassilev et al. 2014. "Why Less May Be More: A Mixed Methods Study of the Work and Relatedness of 'Weak Ties' in Supporting Long-Term Condition Self-Management." *Implementation Science* 9: 19.

Rogers, A., I. Vassilev, H. Brooks et al. 2016. "Brief Encounters: What Do Primary Care Professionals Contribute to Peoples' Self-Care Support Network for Long-Term Conditions? A Mixed Methods Study." *BMC Family Practice* 17: 21.

Rubens, R.L. 1996. "The Unique Origins of Fairbairn's Theories." *Psychoanalytic Dialogues: The International Journal of Relational Perspectives* 6 (3): 413–435.

Savage, M., F. Devine, N. Cunningham et al. 2013. "A New Model of Social Class? Findings from the BBC's Great British Class Survey Experiment." *Sociology* 47 (2): 219–250.

Shim, J.K. 2010. "Cultural Health Capital: A Theoretical Approach to Understanding Health Care Interactions and the Dynamics of Unequal Treatment." *Journal of Health & Social Behavior* 51 (1): 1–15.

Star, S.L., and A. Strauss. 1999. "Layers of Silence, Arenas of Voice: The Ecology of Visible and Invisible Work." *Computer Supported Cooperative Work (CSCW)* 8: 9–30.

Therborn, G. 2013. "*The Killing Fields of Inequality*. London: Polity Press.
Thompson, E.P. 1968. *The Making of the English Working Class*. London: Victor Gollancz.
Toothman, E. 2016. "If You Can't Take the Fat Out of the Girl: The Embodied Strategies Women Use to Protect Against Anti-Fat Bias in the Labor Market." *ASA Body & Embodiment Section Blog*. http://sectionbodyembodiment.weebly.com/blog/archives/01-2016.
Uphoff, E.P., K.E. Pickett, B. Cabieses et al. 2013. "A Systematic Review of the Relationships Between Social Capital and Socioeconomic Inequalities in Health: A Contribution to Understanding the Psychosocial Pathway of Health Inequalities." *International Journal of Equity Health* 12: 54.
Vera, M., M. Alegria, and D. Freeman. 1998. "Help Seeking for Mental Health Care Among Poor Puerto Ricans." *Medical Care* 36 (7): 1047–1056.
Vineis, P., C. Delpierre, R. Castagné, G. Fiorito, C. McCrory, M. Kivimaki, … M. Kelly-Irving. 2020. "Health Inequalities: Embodied Evidence Across Biological Layers." *Social Science & Medicine* 246: 112781.

2 Living in the middle and living optimally

Introduction

There is a strong relationship between a sense of self, our identity, attachment to place and the quality and experience of everyday living. A starting focus of place may help us with our overall task in the book of understanding living with inequalities. Locale by no means tells us everything but it is one way to look at what might constitute optimal living by examining what have been visualised as the best places to live healthily. This illuminates both supra-personal environmental factors and cultural norms, both of which inflect health.

In the second part of the chapter we examine this topic more by analysing 'blue zones'. The latter might guide our understanding of the promotion of health, which is called 'salutogenesis' and the opposite side of the same coin is pathogenesis. When pathogenesis is the focus it is more likely to privilege biomedical explanations, whereas salutogenesis is more likely to reveal relevant psychosocial factors.

Realism about reducing inequalities across time and space

If the 'blue zones' we consider later, and their poorer places of comparison, provide some lessons about health inequalities, then so too do social changes over time. This is especially the case when these are abrupt, as in times of warfare, revolutions or pandemics (see Chapter 9). During less dramatic periods, inequalities in both wealth and health tend to be more stable or slow moving. Since the nineteenth century, Europe and North America have witnessed both economic growth and an arc of increasing longevity, at least until recently when this trajectory went into reverse.

Even when there was an upward trend, dips in that pattern emerged during periods of warfare, with a shift during the twentieth century away from combatant death and injury towards civilian casualties. However in the wake of these violent disruptions, when societal stability returns, so do the older inequality gaps. This mixture of system fluctuation and homeostasis (the re-stabilisation of gaps in power and wealth) has been evident in public health discourse since the nineteenth century. The role of poverty and

DOI: 10.4324/9781003025641-2

recommendations for its remediation have been central to the work of public health specialists.

The persistent health gap

Epidemiologists have used census data to evaluate national mortality trends, predicated on occupational definitions of social class, permitting the details of inequalities to be tracked within mainstream public policy administration (Macintyre 1997). At the beginning of the twentieth century, the Registrar General noted that 40% of British infant mortality was entirely preventable if the social conditions of these births could have been elevated to that of the upper-class. The visibility of public health findings about inequalities has continued throughout the twentieth century. The policy implications centred recurrently on the eradication of poverty and the reduction in class differences (Gibbons 2005).

For example, Richard Wilkinson and Kate Pickett's analysis showed the widening health gap between the upper and lower social classes, which was two to three times larger in the 1970s than in the 1930s (Wilkinson and Pickett 2009). Thus the anticipated outcomes of state policies designed to ameliorate the health inequality gap have, to say the least, been disappointing. Walter Scheidel in his historical analysis points to the way in which economic inequalities in society tend to be stubborn and enduring noting that 'violence has been necessary to ensure the redistribution of wealth at any point in time' (Scheidel 2017).

Shifts in redressing health inequalities have, in common with economic inequalities, the status of being relatively modest in terms of change (although there have been general increases in population longevity over time). Things improve temporarily at particular points and some nations take far more action to reduce socio-economic inequality than others. However, national levels of inequality tend to re-stabilise and regional variations also persist. For example, there has been a continuing health gap between the South East and North West of England, with the geographical divide in longevity reflecting a *deprivation* divide (https://www.kingsfund.org.uk/about-us/whos-who/veena-raleigh.)

There were substantial reductions in mortality in lower socio-economic groups in European countries between the years 1990 and 2010. Absolute inequalities narrowed by up to 35% – predominately amongst men, and for those forms of illness that benefited from improved medical interventions. After 2010 that pattern began to slow down, with longevity in the trend towards equality beginning to stagnate and even decline (Mackenbach et al. 2016). One health implication has been that poorer children today in Britain will probably die younger, on average, than their parents (Marmot and Siegrist 2004).

The reasons for the earlier favourable reduction of inequalities were attributed mainly to reductions in heart disease and smoking-related causes of mortality. These were probably not so much related to policies that explicitly *targeted* health inequalities, as they were with improvements for the general population. These were in relation to prevention and treatment and the *side effects* of widespread changes in behaviour across whole populations, particularly a reduction in 'low educational attainment' (Mackenbach et al. 2016).

Governmental and lay understandings of inequalities

The persistence of inequalities, enduring poor health and the shorter lives of large sections of the population have posed a problem for politicians. In the UK in the wake of the Black Report, which demonstrated that those in lower social groups experienced higher rates of mortality, the Conservative administration of the 1980s simply abandoned the term 'health inequalities' and replaced it with 'health variations' or 'disparities', in the hope of evading the problems shown by social class mortality data (https://www.futurelearn.com/info/courses/public-health-history/0/steps/30346).

The instrumental value of focusing on language by politicians was obvious in this example. However, it also invites an understanding of the meanings experienced and expressed by ordinary people of inequalities. For example, terminology can also tap into everyday sentiments about morality and how those in other social groups are perceived, as being morally worthy or inferior.

The study of the historic and contemporary manifestations of inequalities has been a significant focus for academics, including medical sociologists, economists and epidemiologists. Policy-makers and laypeople involved in health movements have also taken a similar interest. The latter find social injustice abhorrent, identifying a moral imperative, such as dignity and the pain of social exclusion, as a motive to rectify health inequalities. At the same time those wanting to ward off economic destabilisation, are equally concerned. For example, Branco Milanovic, a lead economist at the World Bank, sees inequalities as a matter of human survival: 'The social stability and the social fabric of a society are torn apart if there are very large income differences' (https://www.worldbank.org/en/news/feature/2012/03/30/Why-We-Should-Care-About-Inequality).

Despite these interest groups and activists focusing seriously on inequalities and their reduction, most of us, much of the time, ignore them. Most people underestimate the extent of inequalities in society and in relation to health in particular (Duffy et al. 2021). Also, we are not very accurate at appraising real changes going on around us; our perceptions do not adjust to reality, even when there are actual known and reported shifts in national income inequality (Tay 2016).

The obvious fact of us all living with inequalities is often an unarticulated part of our experience. Perhaps, it is so self-evident that it need not be expressed. Maybe the angst and despair, that the fact of inequality can invoke in some of us, is too painful to think about and talk about. Maybe some of us are simply quite accepting of those in poverty dying younger and being sicker before that.

However, despite these cognitive distortions being common, if they are asked, people can give accounts of their thoughts, feelings and tactics of survival in daily life. People can and do update their worldview, behaviour and social practices, in the face of new information. At the same time, our early socialisation experiences and personal dispositions can remain fairly stable and unchanging. Even if inequality arouses guilt or anger we cognitively adapt to it. If, as noted above, poverty is often stubborn, despite political rhetoric or genuine attempts at amelioration nationally or locally, then what stance should or could, we adopt towards it? The challenge in answering this question may well feed into avoiding the matter, as we noted above, even if people do, in their own way, deal with their social position and that of others episodically in daily life.

Social norms act as components of people's preferences. The moral dilemma element is ancient and captured in the parable of the rich man and Lazarus. A rich man lived a life of luxury, whilst outside his house Lazarus hoped 'to eat what fell from the rich man's table' (Leviticus 21). Lazarus went to heaven, and the rich man went to hell. 'Appealing to "Father Abraham" in heaven, the rich man requested that Lazarus be sent to cool his tongue with a drop of water to lessen his "agony in this fire"'.

In a secular contemporary context, inequalities both exist and constantly interweave with psychosocial processes for all people, whatever their social position and context. This includes, but is by no means limited to, the negative psychological impact on the poorest in society. Instead *everyone* is affected by the shared societal context of inequality; a point which continues to be made by contemporary analysts (Wilkinson and Pickett 2009). This includes not just the poorest directly affected but also the rich and the privileged, as well as those squeezed and locked in the middle.

Today the consolidation of gross inequalities of income and wealth, which has amplified over the last three decades, poses a fundamental threat to the middle-class American Dream (Smith 2012). That is, people can come to realise that hard work and personal effort fail to translate automatically into upward social mobility. This frustration is reflected in the resentment of some White workers in the USA to those on welfare, especially if they are migrants (Hochschild 2016). This culminates in one group of poor people blaming another. In terms of the American Dream, one has patiently waited in line and watched others jump the queue.

Are we all middle class now – really?

Ontological security (a sense of stability and continuity of events and experiences in one's life) is based on having a sense of strong belonging. This can be about place but more centrally it is about connectivity with others. A common outcome of this is that most of us actually want to be seen as 'being in the middle', no matter how much this claim is plausible according to the evident material facts of either our bloated opulence or our abject poverty.

An example here is when a new hierarchical description of social class in Britain, replaced the older Registrar General's classification system in 2013. When the BBC went on to the streets of Manchester to ask people what their class background was, some struggled and had no conscious class identity and some just said 'middle class' (Savage et al. 2013). Today an awareness of say race or gender is common, especially in younger people, but this is not the case in relation to class inequality (Benn Michaels 2006).

Admitting that one is very wealthy or very poor is psychologically challenging, as they can both carry a freight of stigma. Also, in a post-industrial society, the old blue-collar definition of being 'working class' is now a less-evident anchor-point than in the past. Today there are large gaps of both wealth and status *within* white-collar work, all of which could be described as being 'middle class'. (Some of these now even visit food banks.)

In the context of preferred or confused self-attributions, the fact of a shared context of inequality can induce disquiet. People have to deal with actual or potential threats to their status. If they are better off, they might feel guilt for those in dire poverty. Anxiety related to inequalities might include responses of hyper-vigilance and fear of rejection. One can feel culturally out of place readily, and might notice others in the same boat. The internalisation of these subjective and intersubjective processes shapes part of a sense of identity, and who we are relative to others.

Faced with these emotional challenges, come rapidly available psychological resources of sharing a common commitment to the basic need for acceptance, positive regard by others and belonging. We make sense of our social position with more or less deliberation or insight by making a range of distinctions, between those who are like us and those who are not, and signalling this to others (a theme we return to in relation to health status in the following chapters). Value judgements about these distinctions vary between and within individuals and from one situation to another.

Risks associated with the everyday reality of living life with inequalities in health, tend to be played down by *both* those who are most advantaged *and* those most underprivileged. They share the common presentational strategy and self-belief about being positioned 'in the middle'. Semblances of equality, and (unrealistic) optimistic assumptions about the ever-reducing gaps in wealth and privilege, form the centre of personal stories about one's life in the middle (Lawler 2005).

As with the people on the street telling the BBC that they were middle class (or being unclear about the meaning of class in principle), this reflects the idea that we now live in a classless society. This is of course absurd if we apply economic and social measures and concede that the capitalist system is inherently predicated on class differences of power and ownership. Nonetheless, subjectively, people seem often to need to believe that words alone suffice: we are all just ordinary and all are in the middle.

Turning to the ontological safety of 'the middle', this has been encouraged by cultural convergence. The contemporary era has seen a reduction in cultural distinctions between social groups. Elite or high culture has given way to a greater emphasis on everyday cultural practices, which accentuate equality in terms of being ordinary, authentic and culturally connected with everyone (Friedman and Reeves 2020). This self-presentational style of ordinariness is a defence against stigma, if one is positioned at the bottom. That defence is also afforded by the lifestyles of those who are not well-off being subjected to media scorn or 'poverty porn' (see below).

But the affluent, like the poor, also seek to avoid being negatively judged, given their manifest extreme wealth. For example, being seen as spoilt, or over-indulged might evoke moral condemnation from others. For the rich, anxieties arise out of the difficulties in reconciling affluence with moral legitimacy (Sherman 2017). Prosperous people provide accounts, which suggest that they frequently desire to act in good faith and with good intentions. Some are aware of their advantages, seeing themselves as acquiring wealth through 'luck', and even at times acknowledging how their lifestyles might act to perpetuate poverty and maintain class envy.

To mitigate guilt, whilst retaining social position, the rich may seek to avoid the negative personal associations with extreme wealth by accentuating the 'modesty' of their spending, using money for charitable purposes and raising children to be non-materialistic and aware of their good fortune. The counter-tendency for some rich people is one of conspicuous consumption ('If you've got it, flaunt it!'), in order to consolidate, via public display, their warranted privileged status (Veblen 1899/1994).

Notwithstanding the latter tendency, the subjective preservation of simply being an ordinary decent human being can be often found in the narratives of the rich, super-rich, aristocrats and even royalty. For example, accounts of owners of stately homes allude to being 'custodians' of national treasures. They share these with others, when opening up their homes to outsiders. They note the daily challenges of hard work when maintaining the upkeep of their inheritance. (BBC Duchess podcast 2021 https://www.duchessthepodcast.com.)

In this way, the most privileged in society can produce a morally worthy narrative of generosity, industriousness, humility, commitment and determination. Toil, hard work, monetisation and the retention of personal privilege are all reconciled as acting in the common good, by people of good conscience. The drive for wealth generation is seen not as an attribute of class privilege, acquired through inherited wealth, but of youth and acumen that previous generations lacked. Wealth can still be passed down, but this can be re-framed as a perfectly ethical enterprise of kinship with others and an expression of worthy social responsibility (Glucksberg and Russell-Prywata 2020).

The mirror image of the dissonance, on the other side of the social divide, resonates with John Steinbeck's comment that 'the poor see themselves not as an exploited proletariat but as temporarily embarrassed millionaires'. This reflects again the American Dream that anyone can become wealthy with the presence of cognitive devices or rationalisations to account for the preservation of the status quo. This also fits with the acceptance of ineluctable privilege: inequalities are accepted as being permanent and immutable, so we may as well all just get on well with one another in our shared humanity.

Thus, we find a normative social psychology of preferring to be in the middle and a 'cognitive easing' around anyone's station in life. Sublimating one's guilt if rich, or denying class envy and felt-shame if poor, are opposite sides of the same coin. One outcome of this psychosocial synergy is that the objective conditions of the class divide are, to various degrees, denied subjectively from all sides (Cruces et al. 2013).

For those at a socio-economic disadvantage, this avoids any need to admit to victimhood and it preserves personal agency (Savage et al. 2005). Similarly, those from more advantaged backgrounds have a tendency to downplay privileged upbringings and, if the tactic is available to them, they broadcast their traceable lowly origins, to signal that 'I am still one of you'. Politicians of left and right favour this tactic of persuasion for the electorate.

Upwardly mobile narratives of success, 'against the odds', shape personal progression as one of meritocratic legitimacy for the 'common good'. However, they can hide structural privileges shaping key events during individual trajectories. This point about the personal strategies *within* and between social classes, which might disguise structural inequalities in favour of individual claims of oppression, has also been made about race in terms of strategies of aspiring for social acceptance in the face of rejection, discrimination and stigma (Smart and Leary 2009; Friedman et al. 2021; Reed 2018).

Self-identification and health inequalities

Although laypeople are often aware of structural inequalities in health, their subjective focus is typically about their own lifestyles or others, in social comparisons (Blaxter 1997). This focus means that personal responsibility and healthy habits often capture the consciousness of most people. We make moral judgements about ourselves or others by attending to such matters as dietary content, exercise and body weight (to be discussed in later chapters). Moreover, for those in impoverished circumstances, it is a subjective stance that denies the pain of stigma and shame, whilst enabling a retained sense of mastery and agency in daily life (Smith and Anderson 2018).

Part of this mixed picture of accepting, but also partly denying, the relevance of supra-personal determinants of health and illness, relates, to occupational and other environmental risks and the deleterious impact of chronic unemployment (Bambra 2011). Another aspect of lives dominated by adversity is the fatalistic acceptance that there are few solutions to reverse its health impact (Friedman and Reeves 2020). This picture of poor health and demoralisation can be cumulative, and potentially overwhelming, if acknowledged too authentically by victims of social circumstance.

The additive effects of stress, social isolation and being judged disrespectfully are corrosive and need to be defended against in order simply to get by in life (Garthwaite and Bambra 2017; more on this in Chapter 7). Nonetheless, fatalism and a lack of a sense of control are associated with poverty and other adversities (such as disability, domestic abuse and loneliness) and this combination can create a vicious circle of poor mental and physical health (Rogers et al. 2009).

We can think of this ambivalence (part acceptance and part denial of the reality of inequality) as being an understandable, but self-injurious, existential stance. Denying grim reality and avoiding an honest appraisal of how bad things are, is a form of identity work to survive. Positive social comparisons are made but unhealthy patterns of action may then be preserved and risks to health minimised, rather than acknowledged realistically (Lawler 2005).

Moralisations and inequality

If the subjective optimism of the poor, when present, is unrealistic about health chances in their lives, there is an intersubjective dimension as well: moralistic social comparisons. For those who are comfortable and in employment with good housing, images of the less well-off become quickly entangled with moralisations. These include negative imagery about the daily habits of poor people (seen living on the streets or when passing through poor neighbourhoods). Physical and psychological distancing become salient. People living in poor settings can detect this gaze, and this may make them sensitive to stigma and shame (in anger or resignation).

Aesthetic matters come to mind for onlookers about dress, smoking and the public consumption of alcohol and junk food. The littered detritus of the latter is evident on the streets. This might trigger a sense of disgust in the viewer. This confirms (with relief but maybe guilt as well) the comforts of being middle class. The latter identity is defined in part then by *not* being poor, but secure and comfortable, with all that represents in terms of its associated respectable habits and appearance (Lawler 2005).

By deeming the poor to be morally and aesthetically problematic, it confirms the normality of middle-class respectability and reinforces ontological security for the better off. Moreover, media depictions can confirm this class distinction. Media representations shape public understandings and develop the meaning of inequalities in the public sphere through depicting poverty as something 'other'.

> There on TV were the mums (no dads) faces studded, shoulders tattooed, too – small pink singlets worn over shell-suit bottoms, pallid

> faces under peroxided hair telling tales of a diet of hamburgers, cigarettes and pesticides.
>
> (Aranovich 2000)

Apart from these visible distinctions, which mix aesthetic and moral distaste we also find comparisons about 'healthism', linked to class, which is seen as the virtuous sensible approach to the life of 'nice people'. This theme is discussed more in Chapters 3 and 4.

The promise of blue zones

In complex industrial and post-industrial societies, collective living arrangements are sometimes short-lived or decline for multiple reasons. They are usually small and unrepresentative of wider society. But according to accounts some forms of sustained close or collective living seem to increase the prospects of wellness and longevity. For example, there has been greater positive mental health and well-being and greater life expectancy found amongst kibbutz members, than amongst comparative populations. This seems to reflect better quality of life, especially as it affects people ageing. Women kibbutz members report low levels of depression and enjoyable lifestyles, including frequent contact with children (Blumstein et al. 2004).

Blue zones have been identified as ideal types of optimal living areas in the world (Buettner and Skemp 2016). Despite some similarities (they are warm and fairly near the sea) they are fairly culturally diverse places but patterns are apparent across these cultures (see Box 2.1).

Box 2.1 The features of blue zones

'Blue Zones' are five places around the world where people consistently live until over 100 years old (Sardinia an island in the Mediterranean, Okinawa a group of south Pacific islands off the coast of Japan, Loma Linda west of Los Angeles, Nicoya a Peninsula in Costa Rica and Ikaria, a tiny Greek Aegean island). Environmentally and culturally they are characterised by nine common features:

1. Moving naturally (constant environmental nudge to move, e.g., low mechanical convenience, gardening).
2. Purpose 'Plan de vida': 'knowing sense of purpose'.
3. Routines to reduce stress (e.g., napping, praying, 'happy hour', yoga).
4. Not over-eating (the '80% full rule').
5. Plant-slanted diet (beans and lentils are a key part).
6. Moderate and regular wine consumption.
7. Belonging to (any) faith-based community.

8 Putting loved ones first (commitment to life partner, invest time and love in children).
9 Right 'tribe'; belonging to a social group with healthy behaviours (i.e., non-smoking, non-obese, happy people).

When we examine the health-enhancing features, one by one, of blue zones outlined in Box 2.1, they are seemingly small and mundane. Despite this, they are sometimes headline-grabbing and misleadingly referred to as 'secrets' of long life. There is no mystery about these places, instead it is, 'mostly small things driven by the right environment' (Van Cauwenberg et al. 2020). Of central relevance are the apparent positive mental health markers for people living in blue zones, which are mediated by the mechanisms of daily dispositional resilience and a satisfaction with, and loyalty to, social ties.

Another health-enhancing aspect of the cultural norms of blue zones is 'moving naturally'. This means undertaking low-intensity activities *on a daily and continuous basis* within environments in which the inducement to move is inbuilt. This might include the shepherding of animals, the sowing of seeds, growing and harvesting. Also, the fresh plant-based diets of the blue zones require gardening for many hours every day to grow the needed food or undertaking long daily walks for harvesting, relaxation or meditation. Thus, to repeat the point for emphasis, daily integrated ways of living seem to be an important health promotion ingredient here. Rather than the separating out of fitness from everyday movement, moving is built into lifestyles, without the need for reflection or deliberate planning.

The idea that moving naturally in daily activity might be beneficial to health is supported by contrasting examples outside of blue zones (more on this in Chapter 5). For example, the London bus study compared bus drivers, sedentarily stuck behind the wheel for most of the working day, to bus conductors. These workers were from the same class background but one remained sitting and the other moved around the bus, continuously up and down the stairs.

This study reported that conductors typically went up and down between 500 and 750 stairs on each daily shift. Subsequent comparisons found less cardiovascular disease for conductors than bus drivers, when post-mortem studies were carried out (Morris et al. 1953).

When we look at contemporary depictions of the health-enhancing qualities of exercise, most of the focus is on compartmentalised or contrived strategies for promoting increased physical activity (e.g., through the use of gyms and the promotions of sports). Rather than it being taken for granted and normative as in blue zones, or possibly occupationally required outside of them. Instead we find the prioritisation of individual effort and conscious planning. This incorporates aspects of competition, goal setting and sporting activity in which social hierarchy prevails. Success in this regard will be achieved by those richer in resources (financial and cultural).

Unlike the enabling environment of blue zones, other places may exacerbate inequalities. Access to sport is not equitable and elite strata are encouraged, removing competitive sports from the daily routines of ordinary people. Higher levels of inactivity have been found in countries with higher income inequality for both sexes (Van Cauwenberg et al. 2020).

These findings pose a challenge for health promoters, who recognise that daily activity is life-enhancing (which it is), when offering advice outside of blue zones. In the latter, the challenge does not exist because norms of daily activity ensure health enhancement. Outside of them, cultural norms are resistive and constraining. Exhortations to exercise evidently make common sense but those receiving the messages are in a wider range of psychosocial spaces. They are in environments that encourage sedentary living and working and competitive sports are off-putting to those poorly talented.

Accordingly, the individual seeking the health advantages of movement must knowingly circumvent those pressures. Some can do this more readily than others (depending on their ready access to the time and space to move daily in a routine fashion). For those most constrained more personal effort or perseverance might be involved, which might be experienced as off-putting and cumbersome.

Ordinary sedate ways of being in the home, office or car need to be relinquished. People growing up may associate being seated with relaxation and value it as an assumed health-giving position to be frequented. Their environment 'designs in' sedentary comfort not movement, such as in-vehicle seat designs or in the TV room. For this reason, those arguing for the translation of the lessons about movement from the blue zones make the following point:

> By making life a little tougher, you can easily add more activity to your days. Get rid of the remote control, the garage door opener, the snow blower, and power lawn mower. Be ready to use as many of these as possible: bicycle, comfortable walking shoes, rake, broom, snow-shovel.
> (https://www.bluezones.com/2015/02/spare-sweat)

The lessons from the blue zones go beyond this important matter of exercise. They include a wider question of meaningful existence, which we now consider.

Being purposeful in daily life: 'Plan de vida'

The notion of a sense of meaning in life refers to an existential state, subjectively experienced and then reflected in activities of daily living. A meaningful existence (eudemonia) is then a feature of blue zones. This has been explored by Western humanistic and existential psychological therapists. For Victor Frankel, this was called the 'will to meaning' and for Jean-Paul Sartre, our 'life project'. It is about what happens to us uniquely and how we respond to those circumstances, mixing contingencies of time and space with personal responsibility. Unlike hedonism, the priority is meaning and purpose not enjoyment per se. The latter comes by happenstance, rather than from pleasure seeking. The blue zones then seem to value eudemonia not hedonia.

The norms of meaningful activity vary from place to place and account in part for why some poorer countries are seemingly happier than richer ones. An example here is Costa Rica, which 'punches above its weight' in this regard. It is an ecologically diverse island with a culture based on agriculture and harvesting. It is also Catholic (religion builds in existential ordering for citizens). On the island, there is a collective notion of purpose and meaning and an emphasis on finding joy in everyday tasks, as well as intergenerational connectivity and facing caring challenges this brings.

Thus cultural norm is one of 'Plan de vida', – which is translated as why one gets up in the morning. It denotes a strong sense of purpose and a positive outlook on life. Like moving naturally, it is embedded in the collectivised ethos of the blue zone culture. It embodies a spiritual dimension, which might incorporate a desire to embrace a historic sense of calling and a sense of cultural survival or the preservation of a treasured way of life (https://www.bluezones.com/explorations/nicoya-costa-rica/).

The link between cultural survival and individual Plan de vida leads to the emergence of raised collective efficacy in blue zones. This is a product of the interactive and co-ordinated dynamics of group members.

Collective (cf. individual) efficacy refers to:

> a group's shared belief in its capabilities to organize and execute the courses of action required to produce given levels of attainments' and encompasses co-ordinated, shared effort, beliefs, influence, perseverance and objectives in the pursuance of outcomes.
>
> (Bandura 2000)

Outside of blue zones, a sense of purpose has also been aligned with becoming healthy in sub-populations, such as political or religious groupings. A sense of purpose in life is associated with lower chances of developing unhealthy behaviours and their consequences (Kim et al. 2014). However, as with physical inactivity discussed above, a sense of purpose outside of the norms of blue zones is by no means a straightforward matter. Atomised individualism in many Western societies is inherently at odds with blue-zone cultures (see Chapter 6).

Where individualism and social atomisation are normative (rather than the inverse of this in blue zones), the rich tend to get richer and those who are poorer are more likely to stay where they are about health enhancement. Individual solutions to meaning-seeking, at least for the secularised non-religious, are more readily available for those with the resources to enact them. Indeed here we find emergent notions of 'life coaching' and 'life crafting', signalling the voluntaristic efforts of individuals in order to achieve better health and *personal* resilience (cf. the notion from Bandura of collective resilience). An illustrative definition of life crafting is this:

> A process in which people actively reflect on their present and future life, set goals for important areas of life – social, career, and leisure time – and, if required, make concrete plans and undertake actions to change these areas in a way that is more congruent with their values and wishes.
> (Schippers and Ziegler 2019)

Thus outside of blue zones, a key feature of purposeful living is not normative but requires acts of individual voluntarism, at times in defiance of norms of both comfort and anomie in society. Moreover, the experiential focus moves from the oppressive features of inequality in society to one's personal effort. This shift then contributes to a 'culture of narcissism' and a blinkered view about the sources of health. The focus is not on reducing inequalities or finding forms of connectivity and collective efficacy but instead upon an earnest reflection on 'one's values, passions and goals'.

This individualistic ideology enables the person to construct the 'best possible self' or 'live their best life', through goal-attainment plans. These enable them to develop the capacity for desirable competencies and habits for their present and future social life and career. This might involve writing and planning an 'ideal future', with goals to be attained, alongside contingency plans and pointed commitments to those goals.

We can compare this individualism with the original benchmark of blue zones. In the former, a sense of purpose in life is not an emergent property of a group but of individual survival in the face of the prospect of anomie, purposelessness and poor mental health. This is an invented (and for personal trainers and life coaches, a monetised) regime of health. With that comes a superimposed version of existential philosophy, reflecting and partially constituting a culture of narcissism, with a strong focus on personal responsibility and an attitude of 'no pain no gain'. Here is an example of this form of exhortation for healthism, entailing a free self, unconstrained by external reference or interference:

> The best day of your life is the one on which you decide your life is your own. No apologies or excuses. No one to lean on, rely on, or blame. The gift is yours – it is an amazing journey – and you alone are responsible for the quality of it. This is the day your life really begins.
> (https://www.dailyinspirationalquotes.in/2016/12/best-day-life-one-decide-life-no-apologies-excuses-no-one-lean-rely-blame-gift-amazing-journey-al/)

This moralisation works best for those in the social and economic position to act upon the message. By contrast, a lack of control, autonomy and powerlessness is more likely to be found in the poor, as Marmot emphasises here:

> For people above a threshold of material wellbeing, another kind of wellbeing is central. Autonomy – how much control you have over your life – and the opportunities you have for full social engagement and participation – are crucial for health, well-being and longevity. It is inequality in these that plays a big part in producing the social gradient.
> (Marmot 2004)

Respondents in studies of health and poverty report that, in deprived socio-economic situations, they have a poor sense of control. That lack of 'locus of control' predicts poorer health outcomes, such as heart disease, anxiety, depression and self-rated health. Fewer resources are available to cope with stressful home environments or to influence critical health-related decisions in the present and about the future (Orton et al. 2019). This scenario is compounded by lack of control over decisions made by other people in their lives.

Low-control beliefs produce a contrasting response to the sense of purpose discussed above in better-off people. That creates a low sense of control over one's destiny, in terms of a lack of money, information, competence and confidence to control the future. Compare this to the 'living one's best life' exhortations linked to the opportunity of goal planning and life-crafting optimism noted above. By contrast, poorer people have limited options, leaving them with anger, passive acceptance and sometimes a contrived optimism noted above. If 'life crafting' is an option for some of us more than others, maybe other lessons from the blue zones might be considered. We now turn to some daily tactics of stress reduction.

Napping, praying and not over-eating

Blue zone residents have daily routines to reduce stress. These routines vary by culture and climate. People in blue zones suffer the same stresses that others do in other places, when getting by when life is uneventful and rising to the challenge of what to do when it is not. However, the stressors affecting them are fewer in number or frequency. The word 'stress' connotes external events and processes (sometimes called 'stressors') and a subjective state (as in 'I am feeling stressed out'). It also points beyond these environmental and psychological considerations to our bodies.

For example, we know that stress aggravates bodily inflammation and pain and in some cases it is an aetiological or pathogenic factor in understanding physical disease. Those disease states, implicating the autonomic nervous system (affecting the gut and heart), are now well known. Affective states of anxiety or depression have psychosomatic implications and, in the other direction, disease, impairment and pain affect our mood (they have somato-psychological consequences). It is conventional wisdom, with good evidence to support it, that recovery from illness or the tolerance of the pain of chronic muscular-skeletal conditions is aided by stress reduction.

In the face of varied stressors, there are daily rituals of mitigation present in blue zones which might be contrived outside of them. In the first, we find a wide range of examples, such as prayer, 'ancestor veneration', siestas, yoga and taking daily naps. Blue zones are also associated with green space. The latter promotes stress-reducing activities, such as walking quietly in the forest or by the sea. Thus place and context matter in the opportunity people have for undertaking stress-reducing activities (Roe et al. 2017).

The blue zone habits in context can be contrasted with stress-reduction activities taking place in other settings. As we explore in subsequent chapters, high levels of perceived stress are associated with smoking behaviour (including failed cessation), drinking alcohol in large quantities and exercising less, with sedentary behaviour being seen as more rewarding in the short term as 'relaxing' (Steptoe et al. 1995).

The role of food and eating (see Chapter 3) is also entwined with an enjoyable life in blue zones. This includes not just what is eaten (mainly plant-based) but how we eat it. Mindful eating, i.e., being aware of what one eats and not over-eating, is part of blue zone norms. Eating slowly or 'Hara hachi bu' is a term used in the Japanese Okiwana blue zone. This mindfulness extends to stopping eating when feeling 80% full and eating the smallest meal in the early evening.

This configuration of eating has been associated with not having to diet and avoiding obesity. The mindful approach to eating requires a context in which it is *routinely possible* to be present-minded. Many contexts outside of blue zones involved a myriad of current distractions and time pressures to eat quickly.

As far as the content of the diet is concerned, this feature of blue zones might seem easy to emulate. Basically, more vegetables and less meat is the order of the day: complex carbohydrates from whole grains such as corn, rice and oats, as well as potatoes, yams, nuts and beans.

> In Sardinia, shepherds eat semolina flatbread in their pastures. On the Nicoyan peninsula in Costa Rica, corn tortillas are part of every meal. And for Adventists in California, fiber- and mineral-rich whole grains are a big part of their daily diet.
>
> (https://www.bluezones.com/explorations/sardinia-italy/)

It has been suggested that this diet (thought to be anti-inflammatory, with high antioxidant content) accounts for why those in Okiwana tend to live in good health into very old age, with very low rates of colon cancer and heart disease.

The content of this diet has been tested in research, which found that switching just a small per cent of daily calories from animal protein with plant protein is associated with a lower risk for death 'from all causes'. The largest effect was for those who swapped processed red meat for plant protein (Song et al. 2022). This sort of evidence has prompted a partial emulation of blue-zone living in the marketplace of more typical areas in the world. For example, we find recipe books like *The Blue Zones American Kitchen: 100 Recipes to Live to 100*.

However, as we noted earlier, these fragments of healthy living are taken out of a cultural context. In the blue zones, the content of the diet is also connected to slow eating habits and the nurturance, planting and gathering of foods within a wider lifestyle. Focusing on the content is fine as a small tip for healthy living. However, it cannot replicate the synergies found in blue zones of interconnecting social processes and cultural norms.

As with daily norms of movement, the social is individualised outside of blue zones. Within them, the content of the diet is embedded in a range of other variables including political economy, religion and cultural priorities of care between the generations. These continuously shape and constitute how food is prepared and consumed. This cultural over-determination of food production and consumption in blue zones can be contrasted elsewhere with subcultural class differences of taste, which we consider more in the upcoming chapters.

For example, blue-collar workers consume more red meat and alcohol than white-collar workers. In blue zones, alcohol consumption is present but is moderate, whereas in other areas heavy drinking shortens life and contributes to a range of disease states. Also when wine is drunk (around two glasses a day) it is with a largely plant-based meal; it is rarely consumed to become inebriated. Again, the approach is 'mindful and intentional' and the drink is locally produced. In Sardinia, a certain wine is produced called 'Cannonau', which has two or three times the level of flavonoids as other wines (considered good for arteries). Wine is drunk typically with others, raising the next key lesson from blue zones.

Routine connection with others

We return to the importance of sociability in later chapters but it is mentioned here specifically because it is central to understanding salutogenesis. Blue zones are linked to benign connection with others and mutual care in families and neighbourhoods. They are elements that seemingly work in combination with one another. Less obvious than diet, wine consumption, taking a nap or moving naturally, the last but not least of the four pillars of the blue zone biopsychosocial system involves relationships.

They include belonging to (any) faith-based community, which is a recurring finding elsewhere as well (Myers 2000). One of the five blue zones is Loma Linda in California, which has one of the highest concentrations of Seventh-day Adventists in the world. The expectation is of 'a life of service to the church and community'. This positive effect of faith is seemingly replicated in the finding of an epidemiological study of older people in Europe (Croezen et al. 2015). The single activity associated with sustained happiness is attending a church, synagogue or mosque.

Whilst it seems likely that as much as this could be about faith per se ('existential ordering'), it is centrally about the benefits of social participation, a sense of belonging and not being socially isolated. It may be that a synergy exists between existential ordering and the benefits of social contact and its potential for collective efficacy. Social capital can translate readily into social support if a community member encounters a problem in living of any kind. Even without that problem-solving, the mere sense of connection is experienced as being helpful.

Here is an example from a qualitative study of the role of social ties in the UK amongst older deprived adults, with long-term conditions, making that point. This is part of an interview with a 92-year-old woman with diabetes and chronic heart disease:

> R: I'm a bit isolated here on my own, you know? But I don't really see a lot of people. I mean I belong to a church but I don't get any practical help. I just to go to church, that's all.
>
> I: Okay. Well ... but that's quite important to you to stay in touch with the church then?
>
> R: Oh yes.
>
> I: Okay. Well that's a form of support. I think that's...
>
> R: Yes. Yes, it is and the Minister comes around occasionally. And if I needed help I think I could get it from there. I just go Sundays as a rule and then try to live alright, you know, in between times. But no, I'm not ... it isn't that I'd like to go more .... And just now, (the minister) is trying to make money for repairs, so I'm helping where I can there, you know.
>
> (Rogers et al. 2014)

Relationality is relevant to other aspects identified in the blue zones amongst residents, who live in close contact with one another. Putting loved ones first (i.e., a commitment to a life partner and investing time and love in children) echoes the findings of the study of members of kibbutzim. This linked better quality of life in older age to having a family member nearby or being in the community one most values (Blumstein et al. 2004).

Relationality also shapes healthy behaviours, arising from being in the 'right tribe'. For example, non-obese, non-smoking people tend to be connected and happier in their shared state than less healthy people. This social psychological patterning reflects social contagion effects. The latter implicate the spread of ideas, valued attitudes, imitated behaviour patterns and group conformity. Thus, health and happiness are clearly a function of networks that are not just about individual action (see Chapter 6).

Optimal mental health for older people living in blue zones is mediated by the mechanisms of normative dispositional resilience and personal satisfaction with multiple social ties. We will say more on connectivity and strong and weak ties in other chapters – but here we note the comparison of blue zones with the social integration and other places. In the latter, social inequalities combine with a lack of trust to encourage individualistic strategies, which reinforce rather than challenge health inequalities.

Health-related lay knowledge and its potential commodification

Life in the blue zones has the four main pillars of a long healthy life as noted above. In addition, the blue zone lifestyle illuminates important aspects of human creativity and industriousness that underpin salutogenesis and this is *not* rooted in expert knowledge. Instead lay knowledge and wisdom predominate. Aspects of this lay conventional wisdom include the growth and consumption of plant-based foods and good animal husbandry. But in addition to these inter-generationally transmitted skills and knowledge, the routine work involved is central and culturally valued.

By contrast, such work outside of the blue zones is still there but is less valued, with low-paid workers tending to service the better-off. When that lesser-valued but necessary work is discovered to have commercial value, it creates an opportunity for profit-making. This might be something as simple as the marketisation and patenting of herbal remedies and health-promoting foods.

An example of this would be 'biopiracy', where native wisdom about food consumption is captured by food companies. For example, Momchilovsti is a Bulgarian village with longevity attributed to the production of yoghurt. Both the place and the product have been appropriated by large commercial interests, with comparatively little return to the laypeople who produced it. Once something becomes identified as healthy it can be appropriated and exploited and stripped of social context:

> The 74-year-old Baba Dobi has a bit of difficulty walking now, but she is full of cheerful spirit. She very clearly recalls that there were five or six people from Bright Dairy. They left the village after spending less than two hours there. When they left, they took with them a jar of her homemade yogurt.
>
> https://www.echo-wall.eu/china-and-world/off/secret-longevity-village

Four years after the visit to the woman's home and small-holding (in 2012) representatives from 'Bright Dairy' returned to the village of Momchilovtsi. Momchilovtsi had been transformed in the minds of consumers in faraway China into the 'longevity village' of 'Mosili'an' (https://www.echo-wall.eu/china-and-world/secret-longevity-village). The commodification includes folksy unique selling points such as this one:

> The authenticity of Bulgarian yoghurt lies in its variety, not in one standardised product. If two grandmothers in different villages make

> yoghurt from the same products, the results will taste different. This is because yoghurt is an intimate product. It is linked to the land, the animals and the particular taste of the family, and the knowledge of it is passed down from generation to generation, Stoilova said.
>
> (https://www.bbc.com/travel/article/20180110-the-country-that-brought-yoghurt-to-the-world)

What happened to Bulgarian yoghurt and blue zone recipes for commercial reasons is an important consideration here. 'Following the money' is one way into understanding the wisdom of lay practices and production, and their role in the generation of community health. Once commodified and extracted from their specific social context, they are reified as individualistic solutions. Once that happens, then pre-existing inequalities are amplified because of the resources available to better-off people to adopt those solutions.

A caveat on blue zones

Before we conclude this chapter, to make way for subsequent ones to expand its points, it is important to offer a caveat. Blue zones can be read as role models for specific forms of health-promoting processes to be applied universally in a de-contextualised way. This point has already been emphasised above. There is another point of caution. Blue zones might be considered quite rightly as *ideal types* of places of good health and longevity but they should not be *idealised*. They are not utopias, they are not disease-free and some people in them still die young. Moreover, inequalities of status and wealth still exist. This abiding feature of societies is then reflected in the intra-cultural variations of blue zones.

With these cautions in mind, blue zones, along with the need to appear to be ordinary and 'in the middle', noted at the start of the chapter are good benchmarks to think about the psychosocial aspects of health inequalities. In the chapters to come both of these starting points are worth recollecting as we now proceed to examine other topics of relevance to the title of our book.

Conclusion

This chapter has raised two broad points for any student of public health. First, the public response to the fact of inequality is complex and ambivalent. It is both denied and accepted in different contexts and the balance varies between and within people over time. The objective evidence about the persistence of inequality is one factor to explain this ambivalence, i.e., what is the point of thinking about it too much? The subjective response is also complex because it is attended by a wide range of emotions, including anger, envy, despondency, shame, guilt and disgust. Alone or together these are difficult to manage for any of us. The relevance for public health is that we all, to varying degrees, find it difficult to hold on consistently to reality testing about inequality.

The second broad learning point is about the lessons from blue zones. Tips for living healthier lives can certainly be gleaned. However, the sum is greater than its component parts. The latter cannot be disaggregated simplistically in order to create health efficacy in all other global contexts. The latter have their own particular constraints, which will be explored in all the chapters to come.

References

Aronovitch, D. 2000. cited in Thompson, B., and A. Williams. 2013. *The Myth of Moral Panics: Sex, Snuff, and Satan*. London: Routledge.

Bambra, C. 2011. "Work, Worklessness and the Political Economy of Health Inequalities." *Journal of Epidemiology and Community Health* 65 (9): 746–750.

Bandura, A. 2000. "Exercise of Human Agency Through Collective Efficacy." *Current Directions in Psychological Science* 9: 75–78.

Benn Michaels, W. 2006. *The Trouble with Diversity: How We Learned to Love Identity and Ignore Inequality*. New York: Holt.

Blaxter, M. 1997. "Whose Fault Is It? People's Own Conceptions of the Reasons for Health Inequalities." *Social Science & Medicine* 44 (6): 747–756.

Blumstein, T., Y. Benyamini, Z. Fuchs, et al. 2004. "The Effect of a Communal Lifestyle on Depressive Symptoms in Late Life." *Journal of Aging and Health* 16 (2): 151–174.

Buettner, D., and S. Skemp. 2016. "Blue Zones: Lessons from the World's Longest Lived." *American Journal of Lifestyle and Medicine* 10 (5): 318–321.

Croezen, S., M. Avendano, A. Burdorf, and F.J. van Lenthe. 2015. "Social Participation and Depression in Old Age: A Fixed-Effects Analysis in 10 European Countries." *American Journal of Epidemiology* 182 (2): 168–176.

Friedman, A., and A. Reeves 2020. "From Aristocratic to Ordinary: Shifting Modes of Elite Distinction." *American Sociological Review* 85: 323–350.

Duffy, B., K. Hewlett, R. Hesketh et al. 2021. *Unequal Britain: Attitudes to Inequalities After Covid-19*, 88. London: Policy Institute King's College London.

Friedman, S., D. O'Brien, and I. McDonald. 2021. "Deflecting Privilege: Class Identity and the Intergenerational Self." *Sociology* 55: 4.

Garthwaite, K., and C. Bambra. 2017. "'How the Other Half Live': Lay Perspectives on Health Inequalities in An Age of Austerity." *Social Science & Medicine* 38(1): 187–195.

Glucksberg, L., and L. Russell-Prywata. 2020. "Elites and inequality: A Case Study of Plutocratic Philanthropy in the UK." *UNRISD Occasional Paper – Overcoming Inequalities in a Fractured World: Between Elite Power and Social Mobilization, No. 9*. Geneva: United Nations Research Institute for Social Development (UNRISD).

Hochschild, A. 2016. *Strangers in Their Own Land*. New York: New Press.

Kim, E.S., V.J. Strecher, and C.D. Ryff. 2014. "Purpose in Life and Use of Preventive Health Care Services." *Psychological and Cognitive Sciences* 111 (46): 16331–16336.

Lawler, S. 2005. "Disgusted Subjects: The Making of Middle-Class Identities." *Sociological Review* 53 (3): 429–446.
Macintyre, S. 1997. "The Black Report and Beyond: What Are the Issues?" *Social Science & Medicine* 44 (6): 723–745.
Mackenbach, J.P., I. Kulhánová, B. Artnik, et al. 2016. "Changes in Mortality Inequalities Over Two Decades: Register Based Study of European Countries." *British Medical Journal*, 353, i1732.
Marmot, M. 2004. "Status Syndrome." *Significance* 1 (4): 150–154.
Marmot, M., and J. Siegrist, eds. 2004. "Health Inequalities and the Psychosocial Environment [Editorial]." *Social Science & Medicine* 58 (8): 1461.
Morris, J.N., J.A. Heady, P.A.B. Raffle, C.G. Roberts, and J.W. Parks. 1953. "Coronary Heart Disease and Physical Activity of Work." *Lancet* 265: 1111–1120.
Myers, D.G. 2000. "The Faith, Funds and Friends of Happy People." *American Psychologist* 55: 56–67.
Orton, L.C., A. Pennington, S. Nayak, et al. 2019. "What Is the Evidence That Differences in 'Control Over Destiny' Lead to Socioeconomic Inequalities in Health? A Theory-Led Systematic Review of High-Quality Longitudinal Studies on Pathways in the Living Environment." *Journal of Epidemiology and Community Health* 73: 929–934.
Patakkos, A., and E. Dundon. 2017. *Prisoners of Our Thoughts: Viktor Frankl's Principles for Discovering Meaning in Life and Work*, 3rd edn. Oakland CA: Berrett-Koehler Publishers.
Reed, A. 2018. "Antiracism: A Neoliberal Alternative to a Left." *Dialectical Anthropology* 42: 105–115.
Roe, J.J., P.A. Aspinall, and C. Ward Thompson. 2017. "Coping with Stress in Deprived Urban Neighborhoods: What Is the Role of Green Space According to Life Stage?" *Frontiers in Psychology* 8: 1760.
Rogers, A., H. Brooks, I. Vassilev, et al. 2014. "Why Less May Be More: A Mixed Methods Study of the Work and Relatedness of 'Weak Ties' In Supporting Long-Term Condition Self-Management." *Implementation Science* 9: 19.
Rogers, A., C. Gately, A. Kennedy, and C. Sanders. 2009. "Are Some More Equal Than Others? Social Comparison in Self-Management Skills Training For Long-Term Conditions." *Chronic Illness* 5 (4): 305–317.
Savage, M., F. Devine, N. Cunningham, M. Taylor, Y. Li, J. Hjellbrekke, and A. Miles. 2013. "A New Model of Social Class? Findings from the BBC'S Great British Class Survey Experiment." *Sociology* 47 (2): 219–250.
Savage, M., A. Warde, and F. Devine. 2005. "Capitals, Assets, and Resources: Some Critical Issues." *British Journal of Sociology* 5: 31–47.
Scheidel, W. 2017. *The Great Leveller: Violence and the History of Inequality from the Stone Age to the Twenty-first Century*. Princeton: Princeton University.
Schippers, M.C., and N. Ziegler. 2019. "Life Crafting as a Way to Find Purpose and Meaning in Life." *Frontiers in Psychology* 10: 2778.
Sherman, R. 2017. *In Uneasy Street*. Princeton: Princeton University Press.
Smart, R.L., and M. Leary. 2009. "Reactions to Discrimination, Stigmatization, Ostracism, and Other Forms of Interpersonal Rejection: A Multimotive Model." *Psychological Review* 116 (2): 365–383.
Smith, H. 2012. *Who Stole the American Dream?* New York: Random House.

Smith, K.E., and R. Anderson. 2018. "Understanding Lay Perspectives on Socioeconomic Health Inequalities in Britain: A Meta-Ethnography." *Sociology of Health & Illness* 40 (1): 146–170.

Song, S., Y. Stern, and Y. Gu. 2022. "Modifiable Lifestyle Factors and Cognitive Reserve: A Systematic Review of Current Evidence." *Ageing Research Reviews* 74: 101551.

Steptoe, A., J. Wardle, T.M. Pollard, L. Canaan, and G.J. Davies. 1995. "Stress, Social Support and Health-Related Behavior: A Study of Smoking, Alcohol Consumption and Physical Exercise." *Journal of Psychosomatic Research* 41 (2): 171–180.

Tay, L., C. Batz, S. Parrigon, et al. 2016. "Debt and Subjective Well-being: The Other Side of the Income-Happiness Coin." *J Happiness Stud* 18: 903–937.

Van Cauwenberg, J., L. Maenhout, et al. 2020. "Inequality in Physical Activity, Global Trends By Income Inequality and Gender in Adults." *International Journal of Behavioral Nutrition and Physical Activity* 17: 142.

Veblen, T. 1899/1994. *The Theory of the Leisure Class: An Economic Study of Institutions*. London: Unwin Books, 1899; reprinted New York: Dover Publications, 1994.

Wilkinson, R.D., and K. Pickett. 2009. *The Spirit Level: Why More Equal Societies Almost Always Do Better*. London: Allen Lane.

3 Feed the poor, eat the rich

Ingestion and inequality

Introduction

Public health messages often allude to food, eating and drinking. This chapter examines the complexity of food and dietary consumption practices and the way that they are shaped by inequalities, together with relevant aspects of knowledge production, with a biopsychosocial approach in mind.

Fragmented chunks of knowledge are interesting in themselves but because they are atomised in different disciplinary silos, their relevance for particular social contexts might be obscured. An example of this challenge is described below about coffee drinking and its potential for health. Once a particular food input is identified as being healthy (or not), then simple prescriptions of abstinence or encouragement are frequently issued to the general population. However, these can miss the point that food and drink are consumed in particular social and biographical contexts.

Within general populations, there is poverty and affluence and the role of food and drink hold personal meanings for people over time and place. We produce, harvest and prepare food for consumption. These psychosocial processes invite a granular appreciation in the particular situated contexts. These are shaped by processes operating at a macro level which form part of social context. We live in a world in which there is both food scarcity, with its risk of starvation, and food abundance. The latter, in societies where food is available, contains risks of differential indulgence and seemingly paradoxical concomitants of malnutrition and obesity in poorer people within developed societies. That variation is an indication of social inequalities.

At times those inequalities have triggered dramatic social action. For example, food riots have tended to focus on the symbolism of the shortage, availability and cost of particular and essential staple food items, such as rice, tortillas or onions. These have been an overt expression of class rebellion, as a response to extreme adversity in the form of hunger and starvation. Stores have been looted, with points of production or transfer being the focus of such protests, such as fast-food restaurants, and supply depots and trucks or blockaded farms. Human agency is expressed at this point as frustration and anger, because that very agency has been denied or severely constrained about food allocation in the daily lives of ordinary citizens (Heslin 2020).

DOI: 10.4324/9781003025641-3

This chapter then attempts to bring wider psychosocial considerations to bear in a context in which fragmented unidisciplinary knowledge has tended to obscure their existence and relevance. Moreover, that wider set of considerations invites caution about simplistic public health 'messages' about what should and should not be consumed. At times those messages can have a paradoxical effect, actually reinforcing rather than reducing inequalities. Their overemphasis at times has created anxiety and shame.

For example, emotionally driven action, in unconscious protest or over-compliance with the rationality of simple public health prescription, may have in part shaped bodies, creating waves of anorexia in the 'uptight' middle class and obesity in malnourished poorer people, encouraged by a cheap food policy. Supermarket trollies mix anxiety-laden food labelling with the promises of indulgence in fatty pizzas and high-sugar products. The health 'culture gap' between delayed gratification and instant indulgence is as clear in the case of food, as it is in the smoking of cigarettes. Class inequalities are there for all to see at the checkout.

The evidence for what is a healthy diet: implications for inequalities

Food consumption is a distal factor in the generation of diseases, such as diabetes, cancer and heart disease, which are governed by, and contribute to, the inequality health gap. Traditional scientific evidence maintains that eating specific nutrients and food groups and adopting certain dietary and eating patterns beneficially influences health:

> healthy dietary patterns can be generally described as those that are rich in health-promoting foods, including plant-based foods, fresh fruits and vegetables, antioxidants, soya, nuts, and sources of omega-3 fatty acids, and low in saturated fats and trans fats, animal-derived proteins, and added/refined sugars.
>
> (Pistallato et al. 2018)

What constitutes an evidence-based *healthy* diet elides into the moral split between *good and bad* diets, because health and illness are normative. Daily, often jokey, discourse confirms this point ('not worth sinning for', 'naughty but nice', 'I just have to look at a bar of chocolate and I put on a pound'). Healthy eating habits are depicted as ones which involve the ingestion of more health-promoting foods and less consumption of unhealthier options.

Good diets are sometimes portrayed as 'naturally' occurring in geographical regions embedded in local traditions and food sources. The so-called 'Mediterranean Diet' is typical as one which promises a reduced disease risk (hypertension and neurodegeneration), to be compared with the health-denying and damaging 'Western Diet'. The latter is defined by the over-consumption of refined sugars, saturated fats, animal protein and an inadequate supply of plant-based fibre and micronutrients. These diets are overgeneralised misnomers about actual regional affiliation:

> The foods and culinary traditions in this part of the world (Mediterranean) are extremely varied. On the Italian coast, people commonly enjoy pizza, pasta and wine. In Greece, fatty lamb, rice and honey-sweetened baklava are the norm. In the South of France, butter-drenched croissants, rich liver pates and cheeses of all kinds are enjoyed regularly.
>
> (https://healinggourmet.com/mediterranean-diet-myths-and-facts/)

Thus, the conflation of a particular diet with a particular region of the world can be misleading. The 'Nordic diet' may be the 'Mediterranean diet' but just not in the Mediterranean. The underlying sentiment is an expectation that the health benefits of these regionally labelled diets are ubiquitous and generalizable; they result in better health for people independent of actual context. However, as we argued in Chapter 2, when discussing 'blue zones', the extraction of various ideas about what constitutes a good diet and their instant and successful transposition to other places is open to question.

The knowledge generated about food and eating is uncertain. Despite this uncertainty, it is frequently translated into guidelines for ordinary people and health professionals in ways that assume incremental scientific discovery and imply certainty. However, what makes up dependable advice remains uncertain:

> The definition of what constitutes a healthy diet is continually shifting to reflect the evolving understanding of the roles that different foods, essential nutrients, and other food components play in health and disease.
>
> (Cena and Calder 2020)

Food rules might change when strongly advocated positions are challenged. An example here is the recent WHO guidelines recommendation to reduce dietary saturated fats, and trans-fatty acids, and their replacement with polyunsaturated and mono-saturated fatty acids. This recommendation, according to some leading food scientists, ignored 'considerable evidence that the health effects of saturated fat varies depending on the specific fatty acid and on the specific food source' which if ignored would result in the 'unnecessary reduction or exclusion of foods that are key sources of important nutrients' (Astrup et al. 2019).

Of greater relevance is that guidelines are often promoted without due acknowledgement of other aspects of social change and context, such as the rise of neoliberal values governing the consumption of food, and the move away from older traditional food policy norms. For instance, subsidised and free school meals were for some time, after their introduction, governed by a concern with nutritional *standardisation* to ward off malnutrition in the population. This shifted over time to a preoccupation with *consumer choice* in the school dining room, as a means of inducing children to make 'choices' about what is healthy. Thus, even the school dining room is a social arena that can reveal the policy tension between population health and the dominance of contemporary individualism (Gustafasson 2002).

Of course, in a broad sense, some foods *are* better for life expectancy than others. Gains have been identified in enhancing longevity by eating more legumes, whole grains and nuts, and less processed meats (e.g., Fadnes et al. 2022). Despite this broad advice, which cannot be refuted if we see food as one aspect of maintaining health and avoiding illness, any further elaborations can create confusion in healthy eating guidelines. As Michael Pollan notes, the evidence for good eating can be summed up in seven words. 'Eat food. Not too much. Mostly plants' (Pollan 2008). This he views as an antidote to an overthinking of, or even obsession about, healthy eating, which has led to an American paradox: 'we are a people who worry unreasonably about dietary health, yet have the worst diet in the world'.

The relevant point here for living with health inequalities is that the official knowledge about health and eating impacts them unevenly, in complex ways, rendering simple public health messages as doubtful. In particular, the cultural milieu that damns and shames, which we discuss below, reflects in part a source of contemporary anxiety in society. That failure to appreciate the milieu omits an appreciation of food consumption as a subtle and variable social activity.

Advice without context lacks legitimacy

Generic information may or may not be wise, but its application will always be in the context of arenas of social action, which from case to case may be amenable or resistive to what is being advised or prescribed. Advice tells us nothing about the context of its own application, which requires an alternative form of psychosocial knowledge.

Moreover, a shifting social context has added new concerns to old. Whereas food scarcity is a taken-for-granted source of anxiety, what is new is the impact of change in the culture of rules governing food and eating. The traditional and understandable concern was not having enough to eat (a condition that still exists today for many, especially in poor countries suffering drought). However, a different anxiety has emerged in more favoured countries, which is about the tension between delight and disgust.

Eating as a source of pleasure is fundamental; it is not about indulgence but a biological necessity, as a driver of consumption from the moment we suckle after birth. With weaning, we learn to like some foods more than others (literally we develop our own tastes). These emerge in particular familial contexts and are subject to a range of social constraints (from local traditions of availability to affordability). Often the tastes and food preferences established in childhood are sustained over the life span. However, in today's public health context of generic guidelines for healthy eating, those biographically unique and socially patterned forms of diet may become problematic for people. This is because varying past socialisations in the span of the population, about eating habits and food tastes, enable some people to comply readily but not others.

Our innate and learned pleasure in food now sits alongside a barrage of information about what is good and bad food choices, catastrophic accounts of food contamination, carcinogenic additives and farming crises affecting the security of the supply chain. Not only is trying to reduce threats to our health in our diets a complex and uncertain matter, attempts at general risk *elimination* in modern societies is a futile prospect (Beck 1992). Despite this futility, food is not dealt with in a matter-of-fact way. It is treated at times as an immediate or potential existential threat.

Uncertainties about the security and quality of food are a source of anxiety, which can be added to traditional fears of scarcity. In richer countries, these have returned not so much about the availability of food in principle, but its affordability for the less well-off. (This is exemplified by the 'working poor' utilising food banks in the UK at the moment).

Anxiety-laden prospects about food risk also bring with them another social process: blame and responsibility in an unequal society. Who exactly is to blame for unhealthy eating? Is it the greedy customer, farmers, retailers, the processed food industry or the so-called 'housewife' doing the shopping? How do we make sense of these potential parties to blame together or apart? Food then can be at the centre of contestation and 'othering' about blame in developed societies in the co-presence of obesity and malnutrition (Jackson 2010).

In relation to the notion of 'choice', Pierre Bourdieu commented on the working-class inclination towards cheap, calorie-rich, enjoyable and high-fat-content foods, compared to professional classes and their 'eating for pleasure, of what is health-enhancing, and light and low in fat'. Thus, food preferences can be seen as an expression of the larger system that structures class-based consumption, in which 'the dominant classes' taste is characterised by exclusivity, whilst the working classes' taste is characterised as the 'choice of necessity' (Bordieu 1987).

This starting point of the social distribution of taste, learned in early family and school life and often enduring for life can then be extended by looking at the personal *within* class differences and the fine grain of daily eating patterns. Not only are there individual differences within classes but some times and places inflect what food is available to whom.

Take the example of the traditional fayre in the highly subsidised members' dining room of the House of Commons in London (https://www.parliament.uk/globalassets/documents/mdr-main-10.09.19.pdf). The menu has been shaped by the tastes of MPs, some of who went to expensive public schools, where they indulged with glee in eating dishes such as 'spotted dick and custard'. The low-cost dining rooms of the British political elite, culturally replay the nostalgic scenario of the boarding school refectory. Now the taxpayer, rather than their parents, pay for their privileged form of eating.

We see here then that inside the veneer of espoused 'healthism' of richer people, there remain variations of taste. Whatever our social class of origin, the institutions of our childhood, the family and the school shape what we like to eat as adults. However, at times they might be tinged by disgust and anxiety. We now continue with this theme in the next section.

Eating practices and the reproduction of the inequality gap

The purchase and preparation of food reflect both human agency and social structure. Moreover, and continuing with the insights of Bourdieu, food and eating are one aspect of cultural capital. If food and eating are to be made intelligible in psychosocial terms, rather than simply the targets of pre-contextualised public health exhortations, the complexity implied by interplay of social structure, individual agency and cultural capital needs to be explored.

We can think of 'food agency' as the outcome of an interaction between the technical skills, and cognitive capacities of individuals, on the one hand, and the social and cultural barriers and enablers available in their contingent social context on the other (Wolfson et al. 2018). Food agency underlies the everyday work of feeding children, and food preparation for consumption by adults, in domestic, school and institutional settings, as well as food outlets (cafes and restaurants).

These routines reflect and reproduce class hierarchies and often are inflected by the sexual division of labour. The ways in which people of different social positions interpret the meaning of homemade, nutritious and balanced diets contribute to class-based 'culinary agency', reproducing 'taste hierarchies'. Both of these typically alter between social classes and they signal the maintenance of symbolic boundaries of differences or 'distinctions' from early in life. Different dispositions exist about food. One Australian study found that for middle class parents what their children eat was a source of anxiety with a more 'matter of fact' attitude taken by working class mothers (Wright et al. 2015).

For example, studies of middle-class parents suggest that they adopt an intensified approach to domestic food practices, as a means of enhancing children's cultural capital. This process, when successful, enables the child's acquisition of virtuous, varied and sophisticated taste, which is symbiotically developed with an orientation to health. The process involves prescribed routines, parental control over children's diets and the internalisation of self-discipline (Backett-Milburn et al. 2010; Wills et al. 2011). Control and discipline over food can be a 'battleground' at times in middle-class families. Taken to excess it can culminate in the emergence of 'eating disorders', during the teenage years. (We discuss this as a developmental challenge for youngsters in Chapter 8.)

Working-class parents also recognise the importance of healthy eating, but the forces of acculturation may modulate its meaning differently. It may be less future-orientated than the deferred gratification of middle-class family norms. Instead, a more laissez-faire culture may be adopted. This less interventionist parenting about food provision, and surveillance involving food choice, is linked to an affective climate – one that may not always be about self-control for future benefit but instead is about the *current* consideration of affection (food is a way of expressing love for children) on the one hand and economic necessity on the other (Backett-Milburn et al. 2010; Wills et al. 2011).

Recalling the sociological observations made about the content of supermarket trolleys, poorer families are obliged to buy cheaper versions of food available to them in local retail outlets. As with the cultural distinction about norms associated with middle-class versus working-class life, the first is future-orientated, the second is present-orientated. One has a pragmatic and affectionate approach, whereas the other is anxiously concerned with future health and good eating habits of both quality and restraint (Backett-Milburn et al. 2006, 2010).

These perspectives are not simply just a difference of opinion. They play out, differentially, in the moral values in practice in everyday life, as a result of these choices. This then is about food agency expressed as a form of *work*. For the striving middle-class parent producing a 'healthy diet' it involves preparing food from scratch. 'Virtuous' and hard and complex work undertaken by middle-class mothers is implicitly a comparator with those who *fail* to put in such effort.

This comparison might distinguish the successful mother from the more indolent one in her own social position, but also from the laissez-faire approach, noted above, more typical in working-class culture. Both in their own way may implicitly or explicitly consider that they are expressing parental love, with one being about the direct indulgence of need satisfaction and the other about worthy effort aimed at health promotion for a long healthy life. Differences in classed notions of mothering in public are evident in distinctions about children's food between school and home. For example one study suggested that distinctions between home and school based food were more likely to be made by middle class mothers, whereas a more fluid approach to what their children ate at school or at home by working class mothers is accounted for by seeing children as more autonomous decision makers (Cappellini et al. 2018).

Middle-class parenting aspires at times to engage in expensive and time-consuming food strategies, such as purchasing and preparing organic food, avoiding ready-made products, as a demonstration of good mothering. It can then be a guilty matter of inner conscience and a performative avoidance of shame. Such acts are associated with a deep maternal love and commitment to protecting children's symbolic purity (Brenton 2017). This is expressed here by Woodhouse et al. (2019).

> mothers needed to demonstrate that time and effort had been taken in the preparation of meals using fresh ingredients. Those who failed to do so were positioned as 'lazy', thus inviting the blaming of mothers for any current or future health problems encountered by family members (especially children). However, talk from some of the working-class mothers pointed to the unattainable and 'classed' ideals that are set by such cultural expectations.

Subjective expectations can amplify existing class inequalities. 'Intensive feeding ideology' – the cultural expectation that being a good mother is synonymous with intensive food labour – is often idealised through the mass media. The limits of this ethos of aspiration for working-class and marginalised communities illuminate an inequalities gap, which stems from contemporary food ideologies. These require mothers of young children to navigate and negotiate them, and they are stressful. They are a source of potential personal failure if they are not followed diligently.

Added to class-biased dispositions, informing daily living, are the ways in which institutions, such as schools, mediate the seeds of stigma and shame that accompany eating. For example, school staff surveillance of children's packed lunches might expose 'lower' class norms about food preferences to middle-class judgement or rebuke. This can result in poorer children feeling stigmatised by school-based healthy eating initiatives (Inglis et al. 2005).

Class structures impact on food and eating, not just in relation to children. Some middle-class women may strive more anxiously than working-class women to live up to the expectations of food agency. Women in less advantageous circumstances may be more accepting of the trade-off between paid and domestic labour, including cooking driven by practical necessity, arising from the dual roles of mothers and workers, whereas middle-class women may be more likely to signal their virtue by *overcoming* such tension successfully (Hupkens et al. 1998).

Class differences also apply to men in relation to food. Men with higher educational attainment are reported to have greater 'advanced food-related skills', even though they are more likely to have relatively less involvement in food-related tasks. Men with fewer years' education may have more limited cooking skills, but are more often involved in indirect food-related tasks instead. They tend to have comparatively less nutritional knowledge and report more of a resistance to external influence on their dietary habits and food preferences (Stephens et al. 2018).

Obesity: medicalisation and the amplification of class divisions

The personal dispositions and habits of everyday eating and drinking have implications for obesity. As we noted above, the conditions for stigmatisation are omnipresent from the start of life for children from less well-off families, with particular food tastes. Surveillance and stigma and marginalisation start with the everyday practices of eating a packed lunch or school dinner. Obesity and weight gain are merely an extension and expression of the nuances of everyday eating practices. Although it is framed in medicalised biological terms, it is further enhanced with a layering of value-laden terms around the individual.

Obesity is considered by clinical medicine to be a key cause of type 2 diabetes, heart disease and musculoskeletal problems. More recently it has been medically codified as a disease entity in its own right. Obesity-linked discrete conditions, in a bio-medical framing, defy a more holistic rendering of the sick body in its social context. Instead, fragmented disease entities are reconstituted as multi-morbidities (defined as the co-occurrence of more than one condition) which are deemed to be determined by the overweight body. These are graded as basic or complex, depending upon the number of diseases and limitations to personal and social functioning.

The disparity of the risk of developing complex multi-morbidity is estimated as being about 75% higher for the lowest wealth group (Singer et al. 2018). This gap in morbidity rate immediately suggests that somatic determinism is reductionist. Rather, the obese body is also part of a social context that encourages its emergence and maintenance, i.e., an obesogenic environment. The body is a necessary but not a *sufficient* condition to explain obesity in people. What are the conditions of possibility in the population for *individual* bodies to gain weight?

A traditional scientific description of the state of obesity is one in which the energy balance is out of kilter with body weight. Too great intake of calories, without commensurate expenditure, results in the gaining of weight and this is maintained when the intake of energy continues to be greater than its expenditure. This depiction is not inaccurate as a physiological account but it is without context. It is a description but it is a very limited explanation. This creates the seeds of victim blaming and it can obscure social inequality as indicated here by Adams (2020, e1003243):

> obesity becomes easily framed within this explanation as one of quantity and personal gluttony and laziness: either energy intake is too high, energy expenditure is too low, or both. Applied to the specific case of socioeconomic inequalities in obesity, this framing leads to the proposal that these personal failings are more common in less affluent groups. The obvious solution that can flow is one of personal restraint and discipline, particularly for those living in less affluent circumstances.

Thus knowledge cast in terms of physical multi-morbidity, in under-active over-consuming people, masks the economic determinants of obesity and the psychosocial consequences of living in an unequal society. Factors such as levels of disparities in levels of domestic wealth, a sense of control over one's life, access to physical activity and the likelihood of loneliness can constitute a spiral of causation and consequence.

Faced with this biopsychosocial complexity, the standard clinical advice is naïve, as it centres on individual moral responsibility: obesity is simply reversed by eating less of the wrong foods and self-disciplined dieting. Some public health initiatives do address upstream determinants (especially the responsibilities of manufacturers of sugar-based products) but once a person is medicalised for their morbid obesity, the psychosocial aspects of their lives can be lost readily from sight. The public policy on the 'obesity crisis' becomes victim blaming, at least in part.

Whilst upstream interventions appear to decrease inequalities, downstream personal interventions, especially dietary counselling, do not. The upstream interventions that are likely to impact more are systemic not about individual conduct. Take the example of food placement. Healthier supermarket layouts can improve the nutrition profile of store sales and are likely to improve household purchasing and dietary quality. Placing fruits and vegetables near store entrances could be considered alongside policies to limit prominent placement of unhealthy foods (Shand et al. 2021).

In relation to medical interventions, there are disparities in access to technologies that mediate such possibilities. For example, the use and availability of diabetes technology, such as insulin pumps, may not reflect those in most need. Those with less need but are cooperative and educated tend to have a greater access to technologies for easier management through specialist centres in the NHS, which are skewed towards more affluent areas (Barnard-Kelly and Cherñavvsky 2020).

When we turn to exercise the spirit level is similarly tipped against the poor, and in favour of the more affluent, who undertake:

> more of the vigorous-intensity activity that is particularly associated with body weight than their less affluent counterparts, and this appears to be via more participation in organised sport.
>
> (Adams 2020)

We return to the matter of exercise sport and marginalisation in Chapter 4. We now turn to the affective dimension of food and eating.

Adding insult to injury: shame and responsibility in a milieu of disgust

Disgust as a subjective emotion, linked to food, can be transmitted socially (Miller 1998). This can then evoke other emotions of shame and guilt, as well as the moral attribution of blame in the occupiers of the obese population. This shift from disgust to blame might prompt some overweight people to diet dramatically, thereby becoming, at the individual level, a clinical success. However, the emotional climate surrounding obesity is distressing for those affected by the impact of their past food intake, within a historical obesogenic context implicating the food industry and cheap food policies. They may only have the option in the presence of personal self-control but they are not responsible for the social conditions of their own childhood.

The term disgust, in its simplest sense, means something offensive to the taste, when linked to some ordinary bodily practices, as noted here by Charles Darwin:

> It is curious how readily this feeling is excited by anything unusual in the appearance, odour, or nature of our food. A smear of soup on a man's beard looks disgusting, though there is of course nothing disgusting in the soup itself.
>
> (Darwin et al. 1998, 107)

In the case of 'over eating', disgust has been transferred from the food to the person. Bourdieu suggests that social identity, in part, lies in subjective differences that can define us against those close by, routinely or even on first meeting. Social comparisons thereby maintain social differences and can encourage distance or proximity depending on the emotions experienced. Positive feelings of likeness to others can prompt benign emotions of pleasure and trust. They increase the desire for companionship and security. Feelings of difference can prompt caution, distrust or even defensive aggression. We then avoid people on the basis of these negative evaluations. Social bonds, or their lack, are thus infused with emotions and disgust is the one pertinent in relation to negative comparisons. Disgust is the hallmark of many forms of bigotry against those who are not 'people like us'.

Disgust plays a role in the negative portrayal of marginalised groups leading to prejudice and further exclusion, which we noted at the end of Chapter 1. Accordingly, it is a hallmark of out-group members considered to be inferior in some way or other. Disgust, expressed within social practices, establishes hierarchies and sub-group differentiation. This is evident for example within families, where members attribute and re-attribute degrees of confidence in one another, according to the forms of emotionally informed honour. Those respected more for their worthy actions or judged integrity will rise in the hierarchy. Those least likely to be respected might be considered disgusting and these judgements are common at the meal table.

In the case of food and disgust, the performativity in social settings of mealtimes establishes a recurring situation, in which children and parents explore the boundaries of what is, and what is not, acceptable (Wiggens 2013). The etiquette of eating, learned in primary socialisation, sets up benchmarks of disgust, such as eating noisily, too quickly, gorging excessively or without reference to the presence of others at the table. Moderation, precision, quietness of closed mastication, cutlery skills and sociability all might ward off the risk of us disgusting others at mealtimes, and so maintain our personal respect and dignity. Eating has no hiding place, unless we eat completely alone, when aspects of etiquette are dropped to varying degrees.

Within this moral climate of eating and the formation of intimate hierarchies of respect, the image of the obese person can come to represent a history of repugnant behaviour. Embedded in that representation are imagined forms of overindulgent conduct. 'He is as fat as a pig' or 'I pigged myself out last night' are in common discourse.

Attributions and self-attributions then build up over time both within people and between them in daily interaction and then can culminate in shame and the deliberate or veiled humiliation of overweight people. Obese people then suffer the prospect of disparaging social rejection. That moral dimension in daily life is muted in clinical contexts, but it does not disappear.

A label of an 'obesity clinic' or 'obesity service' immediately opens up individual patients to shame, but not the food industry or the shaping of eating patterns by poverty. Moreover, it encourages one version of intervention in relation to the victims of the latter. This re-frames versions of moral exhortations to eat less, eat differently and exercise more, as individualised clinical interventions and leaves the upstream profit-driven obesogenic context unscathed. The daily humiliation of the overweight citizen is now reinforced by the humiliation of their clinical surveillance and their submission to clinical authority. 'Doing something' about the 'obesity problem' means patients being shamed into doing something for themselves.

Given the consistent evidence of the short-lived gains from downstream interventions (dieting), it is at best ill-conceived to promote the notion that 'something can be done' to prevent inequalities in eating, via promoting ideas of choice, responsibility and blame. Some of the reasons for the ineffectiveness of holding individuals responsible is the way in which professionals seek to persuade.

In the hands of professionals, behavioural change techniques may, in some circumstances, be well delivered. However, some initiatives, to nudge or guide people from poorer living settings, may well simply reinforce the negative feelings of obese-diagnosed patients, demoralising them further. The clinical approach might reinforce the virtuosity of being middle class. It can signal a superior professional identity, which is distinct from the people being assessed and treated. The clinician is more likely to be slimmer than the patient (though not inevitably), when they offer the bad and censorious news of a body-mass index score. The latter becomes a sinful stigma that might be cleansed away with the effort of self-denial between clinical appointments.

The clinical conversation is not simply a neutral process of information transfer. A study in primary care in a socio-economically deprived area of the North West of England illustrates this point. For example, nurses noted the gap between what patients should be doing and their level of non-compliance. The patient's deluded account can become a butt of their humour, as the frustrated professional signals their own superior worth:

> You will get some people that will not take that on board and many a time we roll our eyes in the diabetic clinic. This – chap will come in and

> say, 'I eat like a bird. I honestly eat like a bird'. Well, if you're eating like a bird, what type of bird are we looking at? An emu? You know, because it certainly isn't a sparrow.
>
> (Macdonald et al. 2008)

This jokey orientation (not so much the patient as enemy, but the patient as laughably incorrigible) is bound up with the self-perception of the professional. They become the benchmark of a socio-ethical comparison.

Social and moral categorisation serves the function of setting boundaries for the way in which nurses worked with patients in an area of deprivation and also in setting a *relationship* where the power differential was marked. 'Working models' aimed at predicting patient health behaviours were calibrated against their own more middle-class and traditional disposition towards a healthy lifestyle. The latter is the given 'correct' one, or a form of a taken-for-granted and unexamined normative assumption. Self-management is couched in superior language and motives expressed, as a readily available and, voluntarily achieved, healthy lifestyle, through exercise and diet. Patients should be able to adopt those healthy behaviours and, by implication, they are flawed and deficient if they do not.

Wake up and smell the coffee

The main public health messages are usually either depressing or puritanical about what we swallow. If we really like the taste of something and want to indulge more and more, then it is probably bad for us. Then coffee came along as a glimmer of hope for hedonists and epicureans.

Evidence suggests that coffee is actually good for us. In the short term, caffeine boosts energy levels and facilitates sensory acuity and behavioural activation. This can even extend to improving athletic performance. It has a moderate impact on reducing the risk of type 2 diabetes. It can improve brain health and it might reduce the risk of some forms of dementia (the jury is still out on this one). It improves gut health and might help with weight management. It seems to reduce the risk of depression in some people and the risk of heart disease. Finally, it seems to reduce the risk of death at any age due to liver disease (Kennedy et al. 2021; Poole et al. 2017).

When we look at the evidence that the 'lifestyle' aspects of health promotion are often stubborn to shift (smoking, lack of exercise and being overweight), then coffee *seems* to be a quick and easy win for public health experts. However, given the theme in this chapter, the devil is in the detail, if we want to understand the social context of something even as simple as encouraging the population to drink more coffee.

Indeed one starting assumption might be that no intervention is required because typically people *already* are routine daily coffee drinkers. To quote one review, 'Most people start their day with a cup of coffee. Many people would also finish their daily work with coffee. As such, coffee drinking is an important part of modern daily life' (Bae et al. 2014).

This good news story about the relationship between coffee and health has created a whole recent discourse about beverage taste, desirability, aesthetics and the etiquette of its preparation. (Do you prefer a dark or light roast? Coarse grinding or fine? Arabica or Robusta?) Even the temperature at which it is served becomes a focus for consumerist concern. Apparently, coffee is optimally served at a temperature between 155°F and 175°F (70°C to 80°C) with the majority of people preferring it served towards the higher end, at about 175°F (https://www.coffeedetective.com/what-is-the-correct-temperature-for-serving-coffee.html).

Thus the minutiae of coffee composition and preparation is a subject of enthusiastic commentary. Not only has this attracted the interest of those studying culture and aesthetics, medical scientists are also curious about the constituent details of coffee. Here is the view of Neal Freedman, a senior investigator with the National Cancer Institute:

> All of these different aspects affect the taste, but also affect the compounds within the coffees ... But it's not clear at all how these different levels of compounds may be related to health. Roasting, for example, reduces the amount of chlorogenic acids, but other antioxidant compounds are formed. Espresso has the highest concentration of many compounds because it has less water than drip coffee ... Many consumers have also swapped loose grounds for coffee pods. Whilst there are environmental concerns with single-use pods, researchers believe them to hold the same benefits as, say, drip coffee. The latter applies to cold brew, too, but more research is needed.
>
> (https://www.nytimes.com/2020/02/13/style/self-care/coffee-benefits.html)

Coffee then has aroused the curiosity of all sections of the professional classes, leaving its role as a generic public health intervention ambiguous. Is coffee a class-neutral good news story for the health of the population, or is the picture more complicated than this?

Coffee, the high life, social capital and social divisions

With the etiquette of drinking coffee, the matter of affluence versus disadvantage lurks in the background unacknowledged and underexplored in the public health literature. Coffee is associated historically with affluence and privilege. Coffee, within 'café society', has historical roots still present today. It has been a place of performance in public space, signalling intelligent conversation, bookishness and, latterly, solitary online activity on laptops and smartphones.

The phrase 'café society' (coined circa 1915) described the young, affluent and beautiful, who frequented fashionable meeting places in New York, Paris and London. This was a setting to see others and be seen by them. Café society reached its zenith between the decades of the 1920s and 1940s. It symbolised the social lives of rich, artistic socialites and signalled at times the cosmopolitan, exclusive and extravagant social gatherings at glitzy parties and even the onboard life of cruise liners.

That image of public display of cultural status (both economic and intellectual) had the drinking of coffee at its centre. Now it is replayed in commercial chains and the more desirably niched 'independent' coffee shops in our cities, towns and even villages. The affordability of the 'barista-made' variant, requested by the discerning individual customer, is relevant as a signifier of money in the pocket. A cup of 'instant' at home is much cheaper and the ready alternative to the unemployed, or the working poor forced to use food banks.

Contemporary coffee shops constitute core places in urban environments. They are settings of sociability, academic discourse and commercial transactions, small and large. They can be places of contemplation and relaxation and of solitude, learning and work. Generically, coffee is a mediator of sociability. It oils the wheels of middle-class life in public spaces; it is a version of cultural capital, as both a resource and a performance. The point is made here by Walters and Broom (2013):

> The swirling crema of an espresso coffee is regularly used in marketing campaigns to signify intimacy, warmth, sophistication, and 'time out', when advertising products as diverse as apartment developments, holidays, banks, and household-cleaning products. Baristas have become cultural icons and the best are regularly sought out, judged and graded in the same manner as celebrated chefs. Bespoke coffee outlets now sell coffee beans in a manner previously reserved for fine wine, giving consumers a choice of region, variety, and *terroir*, often with the comfort of an ethical provenance in the case of 'fair trade' and organic beans.

Coffee is a drink of affluence in today's variant of the café society. By contrast, in Britain the ordinary ritualistically home-based drink associated with the working class is tea. Coffee consumption in dedicated public places remains associated with a wealthy, refined and higher-educated sort of person. It is a manifestation of a class distinction, similar to the one noted above about eating and body weight. The subjective appeal of difference is then monetised by coffee shops.

This mutually reinforcing enmeshment of subjective experience and commercial opportunity marks off public coffee consumers. They include those who are:

> mostly male, young, work, is familiar with non-espresso-based coffee, consumes a limited amount of coffee (generally not for breakfast and often in social settings), and buys coffee at retail outlets.
>
> (Samoggia and Riedel 2019)

Coffee shops then reinforce consumption habits and their association with social class. They are not simply places to buy coffee. They are social institutions, where people develop (and maybe more importantly, *display*) social and cultural capital. They are a hub of reproduction for middle-class habits and preferences. Coffee shops are places of distinction, and that distinction then is embodied as a performance in the customers who are using them.

The growth of coffee shops reflects an engine of divisive social change. The number of coffee shops in an area is taken as a marker of gentrification, displacing the old working-class version of the 'transport caf' or 'greasy spoon'. These places of conspicuous coffee consumption have replaced the mounded plates of the old places, with their all-day fried breakfasts, accompanied by large mugs of strong cheap tea. The latter have been displaced by the designer (off-centre) saucer, with large two-handled cups and effete, over-priced biscuits and tiny designer cake pieces.

As they predict and afford gentrification areas with coffee shops trigger and reflect higher house prices (Papachristos et al. 2011). This shapes both the class and racial profile of housing in neighbourhoods noted in this view from the online *Anti Racism Daily* (August 2021): 'The affluent, largely white patrons inside gourmet coffee shops can lead to the whitening of the neighbourhoods that surround them, as well'.

Coffee shops contribute to the consumption patterns of the 'new middle class', alongside art and independent niche shops, which foster products and offer us forms of décor fitting for new and educated residents. This demographic patterning is about class, age and race. In other words, coffee drinking might be generic public health advice but in practice in society, it is inflected by overlapping forms of social group membership. Accordingly, any positive impact is not distributed equally.

Conclusion

Food is a building block of health and its over- or under-consumption, as well as nutritional content, affect morbidity and mortality. This chapter has gone beyond these truisms to explore its relationship to inequality. Any psychosocial examination of ingestion habits implicates class differences. The latter is present in both a material and cultural sense. Richer people can afford good food and the best medical advice and interventions to aid their optimal health. They are also more likely to have been socialised to prefer what is normally accepted as being a 'good' diet as a child, which bequeaths their dietary tastes for life. This point applies to poorer people but as a mirror image.

The less well-off are more likely to be the victims of a cheap (i.e., affordable) food policy, which is high in refined carbohydrates and saturated fats. Moreover, parental love is expressed through food in that milieu of taste and immediate pleasure. In middle-class parenting delayed gratification is more evident and mothers in particular work hard to focus on nutritious feeding as an expression of love and a long and healthy life for their child.

The chapter finished with an example of why simple prospects for general public health, in this case the advice to drink more coffee, can obscure their unequal context of application, if we fail to exercise our sociological imagination. The case of coffee reminds us that health promotion exhortations are situated in a social context of class (and racial) inequalities. Rather than having a levelling impact, via their generic availability, they reflect and might even amplify these inequalities.

References

Adams, J. 2020. "Addressing Socioeconomic Inequalities in Obesity: Democratising Access to Resources for Achieving and Maintaining a Healthy Weight." *PLoS Medicine* 17 (7): e1003243.

Astrup, A., H.C. Bertram, J. Bonjour, L.C. de Groot, M.C. de Oliveira Otto, E.L. Feeney M.L. Garg, I. Givens, and F.J. Kok. 2019. "Who Draft Guidelines on Dietary Saturated and Trans Fatty Acids: Time for a New Approach?" *BMJ* 366: l4137. doi:10.1136/bmj.l4137.

Backett-Milburn, K.C., W.J. Wills, S. Gregory, and J. Lawton. 2006. "Making Sense Of Eating, Weight And Risk In The Early Teenage Years: Views and Concerns Of Parents in Poorer Socio-Economic Circumstances." *Social Science & Medicine* 63 (3): 624–635.

Backett-Milburn, K.C., W.J. Wills, M.L. Roberts, and J. Lawton. 2010. "Food, Eating and Taste: Parents' Perspectives on the Making of the Middle Class Teenager." *Social Science & Medicine* 71 (7): 1316–1323. doi: 10.1016/j.socscimed.2010.06.021. Epub 2010 Aug 5. PMID: 20692083.

Bae, J.H., J.H. Park, S.S. Im, and D.K. Song. 2014. "Coffee and Health." *Integretive Medical Research* 3 (4): 189–191. doi:10.1016/j.imr.2014.08.002.

Barnard-Kelly, K.D., and D. Cherñavvsky. 2020. "Social Inequality and Diabetes: A Commentary." *Diabetes Therapy* 11, 803–811.

Beck, U. 1992. *Risk Society: Towards a New Modernity*. London: Sage.

Bourdieu, P. 1987. *Distinction: A Social Critique of the Judgement of Taste*. Cambridge: Harvard University Press.

Brenton, J. 2017. "The Limits of Intensive Feeding: Maternal Foodwork at the Intersections of Race, Class, And Gender." *Sociology of Health & Illness* 39 (6): 863–877. doi: 10.1111/1467-9566.12547.

Cappellini, B., V. Harman, and E. Parsons. 2018. "Unpacking the Lunchbox: Biopedagogies, Mothering and Social Class." *Sociology of Health & Illness* 40 (7): 1200–1214. doi: 10.1111/1467-9566.12751. Epub 2018 Jun 19. PMID: 29916555.

Cena, H., and P.C. Calder. 2020. "Defining a Healthy Diet: Evidence for the Role of Contemporary Dietary Patterns in Health and Disease." *Nutrients* 12 (2): 334. doi: 10.3390/nu12020334. PMID: 32012681; PMCID: PMC7071223.

Darwin, C., P. Ekman, and P. Prodger. 1998. *The Expression of the Emotions in Man and Animals*, 3rd edn. London: Harper Collins.

Fadnes, L.T., J.-M. Økland, Ø.A. Haaland, and K.A. Johansson. 2022. "Estimating Impact of Food Choices on Life Expectancy: A Modeling Study." *PLoS Medicine* 19 (2): e1003889.

Gustafsson, U. 2002. "School Meals Policy: The Problem with Governing Children." *Social Policy & Administration* 36 (6): 685–697. doi: 10.1111/1467-9515.00311.

Heslin, A. 2020. "Riots and Resources: How Food Access Affects Collective Violence." *Journal of Peace Research* 58: 199–214.

Hupkens, C.L., R.A. Knibbe, A.H. Van Otterloo, and M.J. Drop. 1998. "Class Differences in the Food Rules Mothers Impose on Their Children: A Cross-National Study." *Social Science & Medicine* 47 (9): 1331–1339. doi: 10.1016/s0277-9536(98)00211-1. PMID: 9783876.

Inglis, V., K. Ball, and D. Crawford. 2005. "Why Do Women of Low Socioeconomic Status Have Poorer Dietary Behaviours Than Women of Higher Socioeconomic Status? A Qualitative Exploration." *Appetite* 45 (3): 334–343. doi: 10.1016/j.appet.2005.05.003. Epub 2005 Sep 19. PMID: 16171900.

Jackson, P. 2010. "Food Stories: Consumption in an Age of Anxiety." *Cultural Geographies* 17 (2): 147–165.

Kennedy, O.J., J.A. Fallowfield, R. Poole P.C. Hayes, J. Parkes, and P.J. Rodertick. 2021. "All Coffee Types Decrease the Risk of Adverse Clinical Outcomes in Chronic Liver Disease: A Uk Biobank Study." *BMC Public Health* 21: 970.

Macdonald, W., A. Rogers, T. Blakeman, and P. Bower. 2008. "Practice Nurses and the Facilitation of Self-Management in Primary Care." *Journal of Advanced Nursing* 62 (2): 191–199. doi: 10.1111/j.1365-2648.2007.04585.x. PMID: 18394031.

Miller, W.I. 1998. *The Anatomy of Disgustt.* Harvard University Press. 978-0674031555

Papachristos, A.V., C.M. Smith, M.L. Scherer, and M.A. Fugiero. 2011. "More Coffee, Less Crime? The Relationship Between Gentrification and Neighborhood Crime Rates in Chicago, 1991 To 2005." *City & Community* 10 (3): 215–240.

Pistollato, F., R.C. Iglesias, R. Ruiz, S. Aparicio, J. Crespo, L.D. Lopez, … M. Battino. 2018. "Nutritional Patterns Associated with the Maintenance of Neurocognitive Functions and the Risk of Dementia And Alzheimer's Disease: A Focus on Human Studies." *Pharmacological Research* 131: 32–43. doi: 10.1016/j.phrs.2018.03.012.

Pollan, M. 2008. *In Defence of Food: The Myth of Nutrition and the Pleasures of Eating.* London: Allan Lane.

Poole, R., O.J. Kennedy, P. Roderick, J.A. Fallowfield, P.C. Hayes, and J. Parkes. 2017. "Coffee Consumption and Health: Umbrella Review of Meta-Analyses of Multiple Health Outcomes." *BMJ* 359: j5024. doi: 10.1136/bmj.j5024. Erratum in: BMJ. 2018 Jan 12;360:k194. PMID: 29167102; PMCID: PMC5696634.

Samoggia, A., and B. Riedel. 2019. "Consumers' Perceptions of Coffee Health Benefits and Motives for Coffee Consumption and Purchasing." *Nutrients* 11 (3): 653. doi: 10.3390/nu11030653. PMID: 30889887; PMCID: PMC6471209.

Shand, C., S. Crozier, I. Vassilev, D. Penn-Newman, P. Dhuria, C. Cooper … C. Vogel. 2021. "Resources in Women's Social Networks for Food Shopping are More Strongly Associated with Better Dietary Quality Than People: A Cross-Sectional Study." *Social Science & Medicine* 284: 114228.

Singer, P., A. Reintam Blaser, M.M. Berger, W. Alhazzani, P.C. Calder, M. Casaer … S.C. Bischoff. 2018. "Espen Guideline on Clinical Nutrition in the Intensive Care Unit." *Clinical Nutrition*, doi: 10.1016/j.clnu.2018.08.037.

Stephens, L.D., D. Crawford, L. Thornton, D.L. Olstad, P.J. Morgam, F.J. van Lenthe, and K. Ball. 2018. "A Qualitative Study of the Drivers Of Socioeconomic

Inequalities in Men's Eating Behaviours." *BMC Public Health* 18: 1257. doi: 10.1186/s12889-018-6162-6.

Walters, P., and A. Broom 2013. "The City, the Café, and the Public Realm in Australia." In *Café Society*, edited by A. Tjora and G. Scambler. New York: Palgrave Macmillan.

Wiggins, S. 2013. "The Social Life of 'Eugh': Disgust as Assessment in Family Mealtimes." *British Journal of Social Psychology* 52: 489–509. doi: 10.1111/j.2044-8309.2012.02106.x.

Wills, W., R.M. Backett-Milburn, et al. 2011. "The Framing of Social Class Distinctions through Family Food and Eating Practices." *Sociological Review* 59 (4): 725–740.

Wolfson, J.A., S. Bostic, J. Lahne, C. Morgan, S.C. Henley, J. Harvey, and A. Trubek. 2018. "A Comprehensive Approach to Understanding Cooking Behavior: Implications for Research and Practice." *British Food Journal* 119 (5): 1147–1158.

Woodhouse, S., J. Scott, R. Allison, D. Hepworth, and J. Cassidy. 2019. "Secure Base Provision: A New Approach to Examining Links Between Maternal Caregiving and Infant Attachment." *Child Development* 91 (1): e249–e265.

Wright, J., J. Maher, and C. Tanner. 2015. "Social Class, Anxieties and Mothers' Foodwork." *Sociology of Health & Illness* 37 (3): 422–436.

4 Takes your breath away

Inequalities in respiratory health

Introduction

In public health policy, smoking and its threat to health have dominated the agenda about what we inhale. This chapter widens the lens in order to examine living with inequality, by focusing initially on air quality and pollution before considering tobacco use. As with the other chapters in this book, our main emphasis is on psychosocial processes and responses to threats, which are not always immediately visible. Living with variable air quality is a complex topic, because it includes considerations of the unequal distribution of environmental threat on the one hand and the various psychological considerations about having to live with it on the other.

The source of pollutants, and their harm-inducing qualities, need to be understood in relation to the existential strategies, which individuals are able to muster in order to live in the here and now and in localities they cannot alter. Therefore, particular aspects of risk to lung health have to be explored and considered in their situated contexts.

Ways of understanding and responding to respiratory risks

Pathogenic threats to lung health broadly reflect shared air environments, which are determined by locality and socio-economic position. Individual conduct and susceptibility to lung disease are important but certainly not all important. The literature about lung health reflects not just these intersecting threats to health, as objective domains, but also the empirical and theoretical salience of each for the research community, and for the way in which ordinary people respond to perceived respiratory health risk.

For example, if the empirical and clinical literature emphasises smoking behaviour, but ignores or backgrounds pollution in daily living, then its public health advice will be shaped accordingly. Also, if smoking is seen as an individual challenge it becomes a matter dominated by moral discourse for guilty smokers and those around them. However, that individual level focus can background, for instance, the role of social networks in shaping smoking practices (more on this later).

DOI: 10.4324/9781003025641-4

The empirical evidence is clear that air pollution causes lung disease in non-smokers and it amplifies health risks in those who smoke (see Table 4.1). Smoking causes 9 out of 10 cases of lung cancer but 10% of cases are attributed to air pollution. That is an overall estimate of incidence but it averages out spatial differences. Cities have markedly high levels of air pollution, whereas the inverse tendency can be found in rural areas.

In contrast to this environmental framing, biomedical research might focus instead on the cellular damage already present in our DNA, which increases with age. These can then be singled out for targeted biomedical interventions of amelioration at the individual level. That biomedical focus on the body means that specific air pollutants tend to be seen only as a *trigger* to generating cancer, rather than a primary cause.

An example here is in a recent report by the Crick Institute (Gourd 2022), on breathing in a pollutant (PM2.5). Such exposure leads to the release of 'chemical alarm making cells', which have the potential to become cancerous. Seen at this level of analysis the solution becomes one of focusing on a 'new era' of molecular cancer prevention, rather than the political

Table 4.1 The global picture today of air pollutants and their health impact

The presentation of air pollutants in the contemporary era provides a contrast with the past (at least in some countries). The World Health Organization (WHO) currently estimates that around 7 million people die every year from diseases caused by exposure to fine particles in polluted air. Over 80% of cities exceed WHO guidelines for safe air. (https://www.who.int/india/health-topics/air-pollution).
Pollutants include particulate matter (PM), gaseous pollutants (ozone, nitrogen dioxide, and sulphur dioxide), and mixed traffic-related air pollution. In congested urban areas exhaust fumes, tyre rubber and brake particles, domestic heating and building fires combine to create pollution. Air pollutants cause injury to the airways and they create an increased risk of asthma. In a study of ten European cities, 14% of the cases of incident asthma in children and 15% of all exacerbations of childhood asthma were attributed to exposure to pollutants related to road traffic[1] (Ferrer and Klein 2015; Baldwin et al. 2020). Outdoor air pollution is estimated to contribute to more than 3% of disability-adjusted life years lost. Apart from lung disease pollutants also affect the incidence of cardiovascular disease. Because many urban centres in the developing world are undergoing rapid population growth, accompanied by increased outdoor air pollution, the global burden of asthma is likely to increase. A recent estimate is 1·85 million new paediatric asthma cases attributable to NO_2 globally in 2019, two-thirds of which occurred in urban areas. In the UK air pollution represents the biggest long-term exposure to an environmental health threat. It is estimated to result in 28,000–36,000 premature deaths a year (Ferguson et al. 2021) with sources including sudden infant death. There are also impacts on depression, cognitive impairment and risks of dementia.

prioritisation of combatting air pollution. A technical medical fix then emerges as an alternative to environmental reform, as indicated by this heading from BBC News:

> The idea of taking a cancer-blocking pill if you live in a heavily polluted area is not completely fanciful.
>
> (https://www.bbc.co.uk/news/health-62797777)

The benefits of a cancer-blocking pill are clearly promising for protection and amelioration of those at risk. However, it can shift the attention from an understanding of biopsychosocial complexity to a bio-reductionist one. This reductionism has met resistance from those researchers who argue instead that we need a sensibility about 'aerography'. Brown et al. (2020, 973) make the point that:

> Instead of an afterthought an aerography asks, 'why not begin with air' (Jackson and Fannin 2011), being located in a definite atmospheric sphere. This prompts a consideration of life conceptualised as encased in disparate spheres of contrasting exposure protection, risk and safety.

Aerography starts with the environmental space enveloping people in their particular work and living environments. Exposure to poor air quality and pollution causes harm via the passage of small chemicals penetrating the lungs, giving rise to adverse reactions at a cellular level. Overlapping adverse responses include the impairment of airway function, chronic inflammation, oxidative stress, lung cancer, Chronic Obstructive Pulmonary Disease (COPD), asthma and bronchiolitis (Ammons et al. 2022).

These effects arise from a variety of air pollutants, including lead, dioxins, nitrogen oxide, sulphur dioxide and volatile organic compounds. Their distribution is affected by local industrial processes, traffic fumes and climate change. These create an uneven pattern of pollution affecting human populations. Those particularly affected become aware of the impact (with childhood asthma being a canary in the coal mine for those living in risky locales). When local groups become sensitised to these effects, it prompts forms of lay epidemiology, shifting the research and relevant policy agenda from biomedical investigations.

The rise in childhood asthma and scientific advances, which linked small particulate emissions to urban pollution in the 1990s, triggered the generation of more public information, flagging up the requirement for high-precision monitoring and public health campaigns (National Air Quality Strategy Department of the Environment 2011). These included the setting out of targets for reducing emissions and frameworks for local air quality management.

What are the inequalities that are linked to air pollution?

The most vulnerable communities bear the brunt of the pathological impact of polluted air. Air pollutants, free-floating in the environment, potentially affect everyone. However, those in low- and middle-income countries, are most impacted, with 90% of deaths attributed to pollution occurring there. Moreover, that pattern of differential impact (between and within countries) also occurs within Europe (Schüle et al. 2019). Ecological studies point to higher deprivation indices and low socio-economic position connected with higher levels of pollutants. Ethnic minorities living disproportionately in poorer locales are especially affected (Fairburn et al. 2019).

That picture is mirrored in relation to indoor environments. Lower-income groups have homes with higher levels of particulate pollution and nitrogen oxides. This indoor pollution reflects both outer local air conditions, enveloping housing, as well inner limitations, such as poor ventilation and cramped conditions. Given that unemployed people may spend up to 90% of their time in their homes, this increases their exposure to pollutants, compared to those out at work or in leisure activities. This increased risk of exposure to pollutants creates a synergy of health adversity, which includes pre-existing health conditions, chronic stress and fewer opportunities to undertake health-promoting practices. This negative combination makes a major contribution to health disparities between poor people and those who are better off (Hajat et al. 2015).

High levels of pollution are also found in *richer* city locations. The wealthy use cars more often and their size makes them more polluting. In some affluent areas of cities, a high level of pollution has accrued but also those neighbourhoods tend to have more political initiatives to mitigate adverse environmental conditions. An example of this is the Parisian plan to lessen pollution with greater bicycle use. This is the Plan Vélo, which aims to create a cycle-only city by 2026 (https://momentummag.com/paris-to-become-100-percent-cycling-city/).

How have laypeople viewed pollution?

Pollution has triggered forms of lay epidemiology missing from the much more scrutinised public health question of smoking tobacco. Laypeople may have imprecise ideas about particular pathogens in the air they breathe, but they do pick up the difference, between fresh air and poor-quality air (Muindi et al. 2014). Smoke, smell and fumes are important considerations in common-sense empiricism. This visible and olfactory aspect of pollution has a history of sense-making by ordinary people. With industrialisation in urban areas, descriptions of it emerged. Here is one of Victorian Manchester from Hugh Miller, the Scottish geologist and folklorist in 1847.

> One receives one's first intimation of [Manchester's] existence from the lurid gloom of the atmosphere that overhangs it. There is a murky blot

> in one section of the sky, however clear the weather, which broadens and heightens as we approach. And now the innumerable chimneys come in view, tall and dim in the dun haze, each bearing atop its own pennon of darkness.
>
> (https://minorvictorianwriters.org.uk/miller/c_impressions_1.htm)

Other observers of industrialised cities elaborated the same theme and added its health impact on citizens. Here is Jack London from 1903 in his book *The People of the Abyss*:

> The air he breathes, and from which he never escapes, is sufficient to weaken him mentally and physically, so that he becomes unable to compete with the fresh virile life from the country hastening on to London.
>
> (https://www.museumoflondon.org.uk/discover/londons-past-air)

This London museum account confirms the Victorian picture in the metropolis:

> Those born in London were distinguished from new arrivals to the capital by their unhealthy pallor, weak stature, a habit of talking louder than 'outsiders,' with a distinctive slang and accent affected by their need to breath heavily through their mouths due to their congested nasal passages. The skin, clothes and nostrils of Londoners were filled with a compound of powdered granite, soot and still more nauseous substances. The biggest cause of death in London remained consumption or tuberculosis and lung disease.
>
> (https://www.museumoflondon.org.uk/discover/londons-past-air)

By the middle of the twentieth century, the psychological impact of air quality was noted, as the pea-soup smog common in London from the combined effects of industry, motor transport and coal burning houses, prompted the mournful lines from George Gershwin, 'a foggy day in London town had me low and had me down. I viewed the morning with much alarm. The British Museum had lost its charm'.

After the Second World War in Britain, the palpable health impact of air pollution prompted political action. In the smog of 1952 around 4,000 people in the UK died from the respiratory impact. A clean air Act was soon passed in 1956 to remove coal burning and industrial pollution, though motor pollution actually increased. It did lead though to a halving of pollution-attributed deaths (https://navigator.health.org.uk/theme/clean-air-act-1956).

As well as events leading to legislative action, the obvious and tangible threat of thick dirty smog and pollutants provided grist to the mill of social movements for air improvement. This was assisted by communal and trade union campaigns in relation to pneumoconiosis dating back to the 1920s and 1930s. Lay epidemiology in mining communities attributed an aetiological role to coal dust, at a time when many experts attributed pulmonary disease in colliers to bronchitic susceptibility or it being silica-induced (Bloor 2000). In attempts to acquire compensation claims for members of the Trade Unions, officials drew on local knowledge claims, often in opposition to expert medical knowledge.

Thus, compared to the past, one relevant difference between then and now relates to visibility. Today in urban areas, people tend to normalise and tolerate bad air, because it is not seemingly of the same order as the pea-soup fog or coal dust-riven times, known from the past. There is less immediate awareness that anything is wrong to the eye and nose. The threat is largely invisible. This matters, because as micro-sociologists have noted (Scott and Lyman 1968), people become aware of things in the stories of their lives usually only when things go wrong, such as the dramatic appearance in the past of smog in British cities. That risk of smog persists today elsewhere (see Table 4.1).

Subjective appraisals of risk from air pollution

There are markedly varying perspectives on the problem of air pollution which may diverge from the emphases of the scientific community. Most people attribute the key source of pollutants to motor traffic (often with good reason). Despite this common lay perception, some groups can underestimate environmental risks in highly polluted localities, because in the absence of smog, invisible pollutants are still present. Sensory cues, including visibility and smell, are particularly salient. An empirical absence then alters personal perceptions of risk. The absence or loss of positive aromas also influences perceptions of air quality (Noel 2021).

Thus when it comes to consider the psychological aspects of appraising threats to lung health, the experience and conduct of laypeople are relevant. In the first, laypeople may be less aware than in the past of air quality because of changes, empirically, in the visibility and smell of poor air. In the second, the dominant medical message, of changing smoking behaviour, may convince ordinary people of that narrow consideration about lung health, even though non-smokers remain exposed to threats from other sources in the air they breathe.

Laypeople do make assessments of their living environments of which air quality is a component, but how often they are *valid* is uncertain. We do know which factors to reflect on about subjective appraisals. The overall sense of the health costs of living in this place, rather than another, is one commonality. Preferences are afforded by resources to move if one is unhappy with their home. Financial, cultural, familial and occupational factors then come into play to constrain or enable our choices about where we live.

The subjectivity of place then might include, for some, a consideration of air quality. However, it will probably be mixed in with other environmental experiences about green spaces, trees, traffic congestion, litter, crime, or its threat and noise levels. Those living in more wealthy areas of the countryside or 'leafy suburbs' may well note positively their beneficial situation.[2] Individually, they may or may not make a comparison with the implications of living in a poor polluted locale (even just a few miles away from them).

Other places with a historical sensibility about pollution have local populations, which may actually *over-estimate* current risk, as in the post-industrial rust belt of Northern England (Bush et al. 2001). Thus, health anxiety might shape environmental risks being either over- or undervalued by local residents, depending on the specific context (Xu et al. 2017).

Risk judgements are not only shaped by anxiety, but they are also affected by social comparisons with others and are constrained by the vague and intangible character of air quality. Hence the predicament of accurate estimates of risk. Variability in risk assessment is shaped by a range of social factors in flux and is modified by cognitive factors.

For the better-off, living in areas with low air pollution, social comparisons about local air quality might be comforting, which enhances feelings of being healthier. For poorer people, living in areas with more toxic and polluted air, this is likely to mean simply accepting their fate and being 'used to this', just like they are used to a range of other environmental insults. This acceptance may be reinforced by an 'optimism bias', when and if people do not develop respiratory symptoms, even though they may live in a highly polluted locale. If in the past smog signified the presence of a problem, the cue has now shifted to the presence or absence of personal symptoms, given the relative invisibility of air pollution. An objective environmental risk is not often recognised subjectively until people become ill.

Sometimes, people develop narratives that downplay the harms produced by poor air quality (the inverse of the study noted above of Northern England). For example, a study of smoke pollution, originating from wood heaters in an Australian community, found that respondents reconciled the dissonance between visible smoke, and its effects, using three discursive strategies: denial, diminishment and attribution. The denialists considered the haze to be natural mist. Diminishment strategies included respondents stating that wood smoke had had little or no health effect in the past, and that it was in any case too limited in time or space to have any effect in the present. Attribution strategies tried to shift responsibility away from the individual onto others (such as farmers, low-income households, recent immigrants), who were deemed to be the real cause of the problem (Reeve et al. 2013).

Pollution from wood burning has doubled in a decade. Seventy years on from the great smog of London, the Chief Medical Officer's Report on air pollution in the UK in 2022 made the point that the dirtiest version of domestic fuel burning includes log fires and wood-burning stoves, which are sometimes favoured for aesthetic reasons by the middle classes. These are a source of both internal and local pollution. There is clearly a complicated psychological relationship with wood burning:

> The British middle-classes are a predictable breed ... the British have been (so) quick to embrace wood-burners. Because what embodies that no-nonsense, post-war mentality better than huddling around the hearth to keep warm or stacking logs into a shed on a cold October morning? Woe betide the homeowner who doesn't immediately rip out their unsightly 1970s gas fire with its fake glowing coals and install one of these instead.
>
> (https://www.spectator.co.uk/article/the-cult-of-the-wood-burner/)

Thus people can rationalise their attachment to unhealthy habits inherited from the past. We noted this previously in relation to working-class eating patterns. Here, though, the point applies to middle class people, when nostalgic or 'cosy' subjective considerations displace a realistic appraisal of the facts about the risks of internal and external pollution. The open fire or wood-burning stove seem to be the exceptions that prove the rule in middle-class life about aspirations for healthy living.

Occupational, not just neighbourhood, risks

Apart from general local air quality enveloping residents, there are, in addition, specific occupational risks. For example, although smoking is the main single causal correlate of COPD, some workers are differentially exposed to threats to their lung health. Pathogens in the workplace include coal dust, organic solvents, sawdust, rubber vapour, asbestos, silica, cotton fibres, grain dust and cadmium (Sahdra et al. 2017).

These traditional trapped risks in buildings for manual workers are not the whole picture. For example, those working on the outside, such as bus and taxi drivers, work disproportionately in congested traffic. Economic necessity limits the availability of daily tactics to protect the lungs of workers. What discretion there is will reflect status hierarchies.

The poorest-paid and lowly valued skilled workers tend to accrue the most hazardous tasks. In Ghana, the smoked fishing industry is a major source of employment and the product is a common element in the diet. Those at the bottom of the production hierarchy are poorly paid women, and they work directly in daily thick smoke (Becerra et al. 2020). Those who are obliged to work in these work conditions tend to normalise risk fatalistically, whereas those who have the opportunity to ease away from direct risks will tend to take it, as higher-status roles emerge for individuals. Thus occupational autonomy and status are contingent factors in understanding inequalities of risk from smoke together with one's place in a social network and hierarchy:

> women who were initially the most vulnerable socially are also those who were the most exposed to pollution, as they were the least able to retreat from it. This social vulnerability appeared to be due to internal power relationships within the group. The home helps were often very young, without a salary and were not included in mutual support structures outside the family, since they were dependent on other family members. In short, we considered occupational autonomy as an important factor in reducing vulnerability to pollution, since it translates into a greater or lesser ability to exert control over working conditions and to carry out other tasks.
>
> (Becerra et al. 2020, 94)

Through norms of dominance and subordination, inside work groups, those with relatively higher occupational status, could remove themselves from the most exposed tasks by shifting risk onto the workers at the bottom of the hierarchy. In this way people resort to individual strategies, within their immediate powers, to reduce levels of exposure in the absence of the availability of collective strategies.

For many campaigning groups, it is clear that the main answer to problems of air pollution lie in environmental quality. For example, in the UK the Royal College of Physicians recommend a list of environmental policies. These included polluters being required to take responsibility for harm. This requires tougher regulation measures, including emissions-testing for cars, local authorities having and using the power to close or divert roads to reduce the volume of traffic (especially near schools, when air pollution levels are high) effective and proactive air pollution monitoring and communication to the public in urban areas, and tackling the economic impact of air pollution (https://www.rcplondon.ac.uk/projects/outputs/every-breath-we-take-lifelong-impact-air-pollution).

Whilst it is clear that public policy has a central role in reducing air pollution, this sits alongside a 'personal choice' agenda, which is aimed at reducing individual exposure to manage pollutants. Such solutions require substantial cognitive efforts and may induce anxiety in those they are aimed at. 'Protection motivation theory' is a framework centred on the idea that responses to 'fear triggers' can protect against environmental risk. However the intention to protect oneself from external risks depends on a number of debatable premises. The perceived severity of a threat or event is limited by the quality of air not always being evident. People vary in their view of probable risk and see it often as the role of others, not the self (see above). The sources of persistent pollution are systemic and individual action is limited in its corrective role. Finally, self-efficacy to undertake the recommended preventative behaviour varies widely in a population, with the poorest having the lowest levels.

Examples of interventions driven by this health psychology model include limiting physical exertion outdoors on 'high air pollution days' and near sources of air; reducing near-roadway exposure whilst commuting (taking different routes), using air quality alert systems to plan activities and wearing facemasks. In-door actions include avoiding cooking with solid fuels, ventilation and the use of portable air cleaners fitted with high-efficiency particulate air filters. Instructions to constantly modify behaviour threaten to overwhelm the individual. These recipes for preparedness and action on the part of individual actors in polluted environments are poorly adhered to in practice (Westcott et al. 2017).

Whilst a range of individualistic policies are still commonplace they may indeed help those in fortuitous circumstances, i.e., with the autonomy to reduce personal risk pollution. Poorer people do not have access to such choices. Such a policy emphasis can readily divert our attention from wider environmental risks and the politics of their control. One area where a structural solution has been suggested, and deployed, is in reducing an environmental, as well as individual, threat to health in relation to smoking.

Psychosocial aspects of tobacco use

Smoking cessation is a central pillar of health promotion campaigns. The risk of smoking is clear in relation to the incidence of cancer and cardiovascular disease. Smoking tobacco is the leading cause of avoidable disease in the majority of industrialised countries. The two risk factors contributing most to the gap in life expectancy are smoking and low income. Smoking is the biggest driver of health inequalities in England, with a social-economic gradient leading to excess mortality from lung cancer, COPD and raised risks of cardiovascular disease.

Smoking is more prevalent amongst people with lower incomes and the gradient runs in a linear fashion. The more disadvantaged a person is, the more likely they are to smoke and so to experience smoking-related diseases and an early death. Thus smoking and disadvantage are *increasingly* co-existing because smoking rates in the whole population have diminished over time (Paul et al. 2010). The economically disadvantaged, notably, have not been part of the overall decline in smoking in recent years. Thus poorer smokers have also missed out on the overall benefits of affluence, which include alterations in norms about tobacco use. Moreover, those belonging to more disadvantaged socio-economic groups are less likely to successfully quit, when making the effort, and are less likely to attempt to stop the habit at all (Reid et al. 2010; Pisinger et al. 2011).

Smoking is also a source of air pollution for others (passive smoking), which means that in indoor environments (homes and cars), poorer non-smokers are at increased risk from this source as well. The smoking ban introduced in the UK saw air pollution reduce in indoor hospitality environments by over 90% and this reduced the risk of cancer from passive smoking, but richer people gained more than the poor from this innovation. This was because of the ecology of risk: any remaining places of indoor smoking were likely to be in poorer settings.

Given this evidence about health improvement, the persistence of smoking in some groups invites attention. As an addictive product, it has shaped tobacco industry marketing, with poorer countries being identified as new targets for profits. The marketing environment and the neurochemical characteristics of nicotine are the material context, surrounding both current and potential smokers. Indeed, the limitations on health promotion strategies about the habit include the fact that smoking is pleasurable and an enjoyable social ritual for many people. These psychosocial benefits are more salient for those more disadvantaged, who may carry on smoking for pleasure, in order to offset negative aspects of their daily lives (more on this below).

Smoking might, in some cases, have possible protective effects (for ulcerative colitis, and control of body weight, relief for the symptoms of Parkinsonism and Alzheimer's dementia) (Berkowitz et al. 2018; Barron 1996). These are exceptions to the overall harm induced by smoking, but health professionals may be coy about accepting this ambiguity for patients in their consultations. Because of its harmful impact on human health, the notion of pleasure derived from smoking, and even that there is the occasional health benefit, might be difficult to concede by those committed to the elimination of the habit.

The pleasure of smoking may be seen as being little more than an inherent, but easily ignored, aspect of 'being addicted'. However, smoking *is* a form of pleasure and enjoyment, particularly for those whose lives are hard. Many smokers admit not wanting to let go of a habit that is pleasing and comforting. Pleasure is the principal reason given by people about why they smoke, whilst stigma (attributed by others) and financial cost are the least likeable aspects of their habit.

The symbolic and personal value of cigarettes has lingered on, well past the time when cigarettes became linked publicly to health risk, as well as to legal restrictions on marketing and availability in order to combat its acceptability in public life. This subjective appeal then includes both direct somatic pleasure and for some (such as teenagers) the exhilaration of rule transgression. Some have argued that this may have added to the status of mystique of cigarettes: cigarettes are bad – that is why they are so good.

Cultural changes and a war against the poor?

Today the public health messages and legal restrictions have had the effect of reducing smoking levels in Western countries to low levels. In the UK, at the time of writing, only 13% of the adult population now smoke, down from

20% in 2011. The most recent downturn in smoking prevalence is complemented by a rise in vaping, raising new contention about the health costs and benefits of this alternative. The tobacco industry still relies upon the hook of pleasure noted above, as well as transgression, by now promoting vaping ostensibly to 'provide the pleasure of smoking and consuming nicotine, but with reduced risks'[3] (https://www.bat.com/group/sites/UK__9D9KCY.nsf/vwPagesWebLive/DOBDRS72#).

Pro-smoking social and cultural norms, attitudes and behaviours of social network members are relevant to the perpetuation of smoking. Shared pleasure and transgressive defiance characterise smoking networks, and this process is commoner in lower socio-economic groups. The notion of pleasure and comfort are an ongoing inducement in living or working conditions, which are not pleasurable or comforting.

Some occupational groups have been traditionally rewarded with free cigarettes (in the armed services, some sales teams and of course in cigarette production and distribution). Thus, the commercial determinants of smoking extended beyond the actual production, distribution and marketing of cigarettes. It included targeting workers, with the tobacco industry knowing full well that this would increase the risk in society of disease and disability.[4]

> It's staggering looking back on it, but I was told when I joined the company that I'd be getting 1,200 free cigarettes a month, … , I went from being an occasional smoker, a social smoker, to being a heavy smoker because I had so many cigarettes given to me.
>
> (https://www.independent.co.uk/news/uk/home-news/tobacco-cigarettes-lung-cancer-simon-neale-sue-british-american-a8885076.html)

Whilst this doling out of free cigarettes became illegal in the UK (under the Tobacco Advertising and Promotion Act 2002, Section 9) in other contexts the vulnerability of people under stressful life circumstances continued to be exploited. For example, in the US, during the Gulf War of the 1990s, tobacco companies targeted troops with free cigarettes (Smith and Malone 2009). The industry could claim its legitimate role in the war effort.

The profit levels of the tobacco companies were correlated with the mass availability of cigarettes. The more who smoked the bigger the profit; hence the targeting noted above on workers, combatants and latterly the poor less developed countries. As male smoking declined in the middle classes of developed countries, then young women could be a new advertising target. Once addicted, these populations would, as with other forms of pleasurable drug dependency, report their own, at times desperate need to continue. So if the tobacco companies were basically lawful drug dealers, as with all addictive habits they could rely on experienced subjective payoffs for users. Cultural norms encouraged that interaction of supply and demand, so we say a little more on this now.

Interaction between social norms and culture

Pleasurable aspects of smoking feed into the value of smoking and being able to manage the hassles of everyday life, particularly for those whose life is hard. Commonalities held about smoking across social groups include a sense of enjoyment relaxation and satisfaction. Home is a place where smoking is associated with privacy and comfort. Those who smoke feel that they are judged negatively and looked down upon publicly, creating feelings of constraint.

There are a number of studies that explore the reception and uptake of smoking cessation measures and bans, 'where the social unacceptability of smoking has dramatically increased, there is an inverse association between conscientiousness and smoking status' (Lee et al. 2020). There is evidence for targeted interventions oriented to marginalised groups (e.g., psychiatric patients), which have some short-term effects but the pattern of persistence in poorer groups remains (Gilbody et al. 2019; Aschbrenner et al. 2019).

The value and status linked to early smoking represent an important psychological prop and identity for future smoking practices. Older smokers view the habit nostalgically, as something valued in their youth as 'cool' and sophisticated (Paul et al. 2010). Young smokers are seemingly more accepting of legislation; older people less so and they are more likely to consider it an erosion of their rights. Weight control has been seen as a reason for continuing to smoke amongst women but not men. Thus several social variables (in this case age and sex) are relevant, even if social class remains the dominant predictor of smoking patterns in society.

People living in disadvantaged circumstances might use smoking as a bid to resist the stigma and shame of poverty and poor health and to (re)assert individual agency and control, by continuing to smoke. Smoking has been found to be a prop in the worlds of young poorer women, who have more caring responsibilities and multiple daily challenges. Cigarette smoking can act as a coping strategy, in the face of the stresses of poverty and caring roles, as Hilary Graham noted here:

> poverty and caring combine with low levels of physical and emotional energy, with sleep problems and with feelings of social isolation. In this context, smoking appeared to provide a way of coping with caring-in-poverty: a way of coping alone with the demands of full-time caring and with the struggle of making ends meet.
>
> (Graham 1987, 47)

Despite awareness of the health risks of the habit, a smoking identity connects people with peers. The narrative amongst a shared network can depict smoking and its effects fatalistically, as one amongst many risks in the lives of multiple disadvantages, so smoking in peer groups can be viewed and experienced as a source of solidarity, forbearance and connectivity (Hiscock et al. 2012).

Networks influence *both* the cessation *and* continuation of smoking habits. Policies on smoking restriction, in bars, restaurants and office-working, have encouraged the first network tendency, and delimited the second. Seeing and being with others smoking in public indicates a 'permission' to smoke. The more normative it is to smoke at home the more others are inclined to do likewise. Social network barriers to stopping smoking include the transmission of pro-smoking social norms and practices of social network members. Quitting together with other network members entails being able to model a cessation role model in one's network, as well as being in receipt of direct encouragement and affirmation from other network members, who are also trying to give up smoking (Ashbrenner et al. 2019).

A study about class attitudes to smoking cessation found that those from lower socio-economic groupings saw being persuaded to give up as potential erosion of previously held 'rights', which would need to be replaced in some way or other by government. This contrasts with smoking restrictions being seen as beneficial and an aid to quitting amongst middle-class respondents. Continuing to smoke in this group came with a sense of condemnation and censure. Risking alienation and ostracisation from continuing to smoke invoked shamed caution, such as having to be a 'clean' smoker and not someone who smokes near others or inside. Smoking was seen as a hidden activity, when one has to leave a group or situation to smoke. This can trigger a sense of exclusion and feelings of 'idiocy' and from being seen as unable to look after oneself. There is also a heightened awareness of anti-smoking pressures in the workplace in this scorned outgroup (Paul et al. 2010).

Thus, when we come to unpick the psychosocial complexity of smoking cessation and continuation, considerations of class and different moral stances emerge. Those who are less well-off are perhaps more defiant, in the face of a loss of a valued prop and source of sociability and belonging. Some studies even suggest that the capacity to desist from smoking represents a form of individual conscientiousness, which is then class-linked (as in other psychological attributions such as intelligence) (Lee et al. 2002). Smokers knowing their stigmatised position may then, in a state of guilt or shame, actually avoid help to stop (Christakis and Fowler 2008). This creates a spiral of poorer smokers being doubly stigmatised by their better-off peers, as both a health burden and a moral failure.

In terms of quitting attempts, smokers in poorer groups are more vulnerable to relapse. This has been attributed to having higher nicotine dependence, lower self-efficacy and less success when attempting to quit than more advantaged groups. Smokers in the low socio-economic group are more likely to report attempts as a negative experience. They report being more likely to feel depressed, restless and anxious (Pisinger et al. 2011; Hiscock et al. 2011; Boland et al. 2017). Targeted interventions at less well-off smoking groups tried in the past show effectiveness but quitting effects were short-lived, which might suggest the strong enduring pull of cultural and local network effects and inadequacy of nicotine replacement therapy as a substitute for smoking cigarettes (Lucherini et al. 2020). In other words, if smoking remains highly prevalent in an immediate peer network, then the default to returning to the habit is more likely than when the majority in a network are non-smokers.

This pessimistic picture about quitting in poorer populations may mean that greater hopes lie in prevention options, such as altering the norms of children in schools. Primary socialisation can alter network norms, whereas secondary socialisation (learning how to be a non-smoker) is always rubbing up against the power and inertia of immediate normativity and social contagion, in particular cultural settings. Prospects for such a shift are undermined, whilst ever poverty exists and it encourages fatalistic defiance. It may be that using properties of social networks identified as being related to smoking such as opportunities for social comparison and role modelling and support from peers of similar backgrounds together with addressing poverty, would have more success (Landais et al. 2012).

Finally it is worth mentioning vaping, which has a contradictory and uncertain potential as a possible tool in inequalities in smoking cessation. Recently it has been promoted as a smoking cessation method, with the NHS in the UK offering incentives. This implies that policymakers are proposing that is a less harmful alternative to smoking.

However, at the time of writing this rationale remains contested. The nicotine in vaping still has detrimental cardiovascular effects. Also adopting vaping at a young age, in those who are not yet smokers may simply reproduce a health inequality (if poorer children adopt the habit more). Yet it may also present the introduction of a new source of harm compared to not smoking. Inequalities in vaping amongst never-smoking youth and adult ex-smokers, suggest the potential widening of health inequalities. But given that poorer people are more likely to relapse when trying to quit smoking, vaping might enable that group in particular to eventually stop (Green et al. 2020). Vaping remains an ambiguous prospect for improved lung health in the population and that ambiguity applies to its implications for inequality.

Conclusion

This chapter has examined some nuances of air and lung health. Smoking cessation has predominated in public health campaigns. However, the seemingly self-evident political centrality of smoking, for policy-makers and clinicians, may encourage us to suspend criticality about the wider context of breathing. When we address that wider context, we encounter obdurate social determinants of poor air quality, which invite our understanding of distal commercial interests on the one hand and proximate personal responses on the other. Both of these reflect social conditions and personal interests.

During the twentieth century the mode of production under industrial capitalism (and state socialism) generated pollution. The internal combustion engine during the same period amplified this trend. Pollutants enveloped the whole population but they disproportionately affected the poor, with implications for the uneven distribution of both morbidity and mortality.

Post-industrial areas in Western societies, though aesthetically still scarred ('the rust belt') are now less polluted than in the past, whereas older more agrarian societies, with increased motor traffic, are witnessing increases in poor air quality with economic development. Apart from the differential health impact across the world, this changing pattern has implications for the survival of the human species, not merely its current living members, because of the climate change it has triggered.

If the structural inequalities expose the poor to greater environmental risk in the home and workplace, then their options for self-protection are also more limited than for the better-off. Moreover, a central threat to lung health, cigarette smoking, is both a stigmatised coping habit and one that has been encouraged disproportionately in some working environments. Central to compliance and resistance to tobacco use are relationships. These are a vehicle for solidarity in the poor, and desistance in the better-off.

When we considered air quality in the first part of the chapter, it became obvious that indoor and outdoor pollution is a shared threat to health for all. However, better-off people have more opportunities to live and work in healthier environments. This affords them greater access to health-enhancing habits. Thus, the link between air quality, tobacco use and human health requires a biopsychosocial sensibility and much of our understanding remains rudimentary, especially in relation to subjective mediations, in particular times and places.

References

Ammons, S., H. Aja, A.A. Ghazarian, et al. 2022. "Perception of Worry of Harm From Air Pollution: Results from the Health Information National Trends Survey (Hints)." *BMC Public Health* 22 (1): 1254.

Aschbrenner, K.A., J.A. Naslund, L. Gill, L., Hughes, T., O'Malley, A.J., Bartels, S.J., and Brunette, M.F. 2019. "Qualitative Analysis of Social Network Influences on Quitting Smoking Among Individuals with Serious Mental Illness." *Journal of Mental Health* 28 (5): 475–481.

Baldwin, C., B. Cave, and P. Rawstorne 2020. "Measuring the Impact of Public Understandings of Risk from Urban and Industrial Development on Community Psychosocial Well-Being: A Mixed Methods Strategy." *International Journal of Community Well-Being* 3 (1): 57–82.

Baron, J.A. 1996. "Beneficial Effects of Nicotine and Cigarette Smoking: The Real, The Possible and the Spurious." *British Medical Bulletin* 52 (1): 58–73.

Becerra, S., M. Belland, A. Bonnassieux, and C. Liousse. (2020). "'Living with' Air Pollution in Abidjan (Cote d'Ivoire): A Study of Risk Culture and Silent

Suffering in Three Occupational Areas." *Health, Risk & Society* 22 (1): 86–106.

Berkowitz, L., B.M. Schultz, G.A. Salazar, C. Pardo-Roa, V.P. Sebastián, M.M. Álvarez-Lobos, and S.M. Bueno. 2018."Impact of Cigarette Smoking on the Gastrointestinal Tract Inflammation: Opposing Effects in Crohn's Disease and Ulcerative Colitis." *Frontiers in Immunology* 9: 74.

Bloor, M. 2000. "The South Wales Miners Federation, Miners' Lung and the Instrumental Use of Expertise, 1900–1950." *Social Studies of Science* 30 (1): 125–140. doi: 10.1177/030631200030001005.

Boland, V.C., R.P. Mattick, H. McRobbie, et al. 2017. "'*I'm Not Strong Enough; I'm Not Good Enough. I Can't Do This, I'm Failing*': A Qualitative Study of Low-Socioeconomic Status Smokers' Experiences with Accessing Cessation Support and the Role for Alternative Technology-Based Support." *International Journal Equity Health* 16 (1): 196.

Brown, N., C. Buse, A. Lewis, D. Martin, and S. Nettleton. 2020. "Air Care: An 'Aerography' of Breath, Buildings and Bugs in the Cystic Fibrosis Clinic." *Sociology of Health & Illness* 42 (5): 972–986.

Bush, J., S. Moffatt, and C. Dunn. 2001. "'Even the Birds Round Here Cough': Stigma, Air Pollution and Health in Teesside." *Health & Place* 7 (1): 47–56.

Christakis, N.A., and J.H. Fowler. 2008. "The Collective Dynamics of Smoking in a Large Social Network." *New England Journal of Medicine* 358 (21): 2249–2258.

Fairburn, J., S.A. Schüle, S. Dreger, L. Karla Hilz, and G. Bolte. 2019. "Social Inequalities in Exposure to Ambient Air Pollution: A Systematic Review in the Who European Region." *International Journal of Environmental Research & Public Health* 16 (17): 3127.

Ferguson, L., J. Taylor, K. Zhou, et al. 2021. "Systemic Inequalities in Indoor Air Pollution Exposure in London, UK." *BuildCities* 2 (1): 425–448.

Ferrer, R., and W.M. Klein. 2015. "Risk Perceptions and Health Behavior." *Current Opinion in Psychology* 5: 85–89.

Gilbody, S., E. Peckham, D. Bailey, et al. 2019. "Smoking Cessation for People with Severe Mental Illness (Scimitar+): A Pragmatic Randomised Controlled Trial." *Lancet Psychiatry* 6 (5): 379–390.

Gourd, E. 2022. "New Evidence That Air Pollution Contributes Substantially to Lung Cancer." *Lancet Oncology* 23 (10): e448.

Graham, H. 1987. "Women's Smoking and Family Health." *Social Science & Medicine* 25 (1): 47–56.

Green, M.J., L. Gray, H. Sweeting, and M. Benzeval. 2020. "Socioeconomic Patterning of Vaping By Smoking Status Among UK Adults and Youth." *BMC Public Health* 20 (1): 183.

Hajat, A., C. Hsia, and M.S. O'Neill. 2015. "Socioeconomic Disparities and Air Pollution Exposure: A Global Review." *Current Environmental Health Reports* 2 (4): 440–450.

Hiscock, R., K. Judge, and L. Bauld. 2011. "Social Inequalities in Quitting Smoking: What Factors Mediate The Relationship Between Socioeconomic Position and Smoking Cessation?" *Journal of Public Health* 33 (1): 39–47.

Hiscock, R., L. Bauld, A. Amos, and S. Platt. 2012. "Smoking and Socioeconomic Status in England: The Rise of the Never Smoker and the Disadvantaged Smoker." *Journal of Public Health* 34 (3): 390–396.

Jackson, M., and M. Fannin. 2011. "Letting Georgraphy Fall Where It May - Aerographies Address the Elemental." *Environmental and Planning* 29 (1): 435–444.

Lucherini, M., S. Hill, and K. Smith. 2020. "Inequalities, Harm Reduction and Non-Combustible Nicotine Products: A Meta-Ethnography of Qualitative Evidence." *BMC Public Health* 20 (1): 943.

Lee, C., M. Gao, and C.D. Ryff. 2002. "Conscientiousness and Smoking: Do Cultural Context and Gender Matter?" *Frontiers in Psychology* 11: 1593.

Lee, K.K., R. Bing, J. Kiang, J., S. Bashir, et al. 2020. "Adverse Health Effects Associated with Household Air Pollution: A Systematic Review, Meta-Analysis, and Burden Estimation Study." *Lancet. Global Health*, 8 (11): e1427–e1434.

Landais, L.L., E.C. van Wijk, and J. Harting. 2012. "Smoking Cessation in Lower Socioeconomic Groups: Adaptation and Pilot Test of a Rolling Group Intervention." *Biomedical Research International* 2021: 8830912.

Muindi, K., T. Egondi, E. Kimani-Murage, J. Rocklov, and N. Ng. 2014. "'We Are Used to This': A Qualitative Assessment of the Perceptions of and Attitudes Towards Air Pollution Amongst Slum Residents in Nairobi." *BMC Public Health* 14: 226.

Noël, C., C. Vanroelen, and S. Gadeyne. 2021. "Qualitative Research About Public Health Risk Perceptions on Ambient Air Pollution. A Review Study." *Social Science & Medicine: Population HealthSSM – Population Health* 15: 100879.

Paul, C.L., S. Ross, J. Bryant, et al. 2010. "The Social Context of Smoking: A Qualitative Study Comparing Smokers of High Versus Low Socioeconomic Position." *BMC Public Health* 10: 211.

Pisinger, C., M. Aadahl, U. Toft, and T. Jørgensen. 2011. "Motives to Quit Smoking And Reasons to Relapse Differ By Socioeconomic Status." *Preventative Medicine* 52 (1): 48–52.

Reeve, I., J. Scott, D. Hine et al., 2013. "'This Is Not a Burning Issue for Me': How Citizens Justify Their Use of Wood Heaters in a City with Severe Air Pollution Problem." *Energy Policy* 57 (June): 204–211.

Reid, J.L., D. Hammond, C. Boudreau, G.T. Fong, and M. Siahpush. 2010. "ITC Collaboration. Socioeconomic Disparities in Quit Intentions, Quit Attempts, and Smoking Abstinence Among Smokers in Four Western Countries: Findings from the International Tobacco Control Four Country Survey." *Nicotine & Tobacco Research* 12 (Suppl 1): S20–S33.

Sadhra, S., O.P. Kurmi, S.S. Sadhra, K.B. Lam, and J.G. Ayres. 2017. "Occupational COPD and Job Exposure Matrices: A Systematic Review and Meta-Analysis." *International Journal of Chronic Obstructive Pulmonary Disease* 12: 725–734.

Schüle, S.A., S. Dreger, L. Karla Hilz, and G. Bolte. 2019. "Social Inequalities in Exposure to Ambient Air Pollution: A Systematic Review in the WHO European Region." *International Journal of Environmental Research & Public Health* 16 (17): 3127.

Scott, M.B., and S.M. Lyman. 1968. "Accounts." *American Journal of Sociology* 33 (1): 12–18.

Smith, E.A., and R.E. Malone2009. "'Everywhere the Soldier Will Be': Wartime Tobacco Promotion in the US Military." *American Journal of Public Health* 99 (9): 1595–1602.

The air quality strategy for England, Scotland, Wales and Northern Ireland policy paper. 2011. Department of Environment Food and Rural Affairs Uk Gov.

Westcott, R., K. Ronan, H. Bambrick, et al. 2017. "Expanding Protection Motivation Theory: Investigating an Application to Animal Owners and Emergency Responders in Bushfire Emergencies." *BMC Psychology* 5 (1): 13.

Xu, J., C.S.F. Chi, and K. Zhu. 2017. "Concern or Apathy: The Attitude of the Public Toward Urban Air Pollution." *Journal of Risk Research* 20 (4): 482–498.

5 Running up that hill

Living unequally with the meaning of sport and exercise

Introduction

Inactivity levels are patterned by socio-economic disparities. A lack of exercise is implicated in a range of health conditions including obesity, cardiovascular problems, cancer and type 2 diabetes (Wilmot et al. 2012). Exercise is imbued with preventative powers in the young, those in vulnerable middle age and those who are older already suffering from long-term conditions. This is partly about physiological efficiency preventing ill health and aiding recovery from injury or illness and partly about improving self-image for all these groups (Wankel and Burger 1990).

The public health challenge of being sedentary is typically framed as being a matter of 'lifestyle'. However, this may mask the subtleties and variations that come with socio-cultural context and identity, which lay beyond 'the choices' made by individuals. Access to activities varies according to location, as well as learned expectations about exercise. Engaging in physical activity is a matter of practicality and culture, symbolically reflecting socio-marginalisation or inclusion, as well as class, ethnic and sex differences. The symbolic duality of exercise (as a matter of *both* health *and* one of cultural distinction), places individual agency centre stage. Whether it is to stave off death, maintain bodily health or signal status, individuals must, according to normative messages, take responsibility for their bodies, via exercise.

As a social activity, particular cultural ideas and practices about exercise are transmitted between people. These are products of a 'hidden curriculum' of distinctions and differences that have a moral currency. Exercise is taken for granted as a virtuous activity, with the vice of indolence or sloth being implied by its opposite. This has implications for social comparisons. Participating in exercise involves social performativity, picked up by mimicry and modelling, on the pitch or in the park or the gym. Some forms of exercise might cause personal demoralisation and a sense of social defeat for those who lack the confidence, ability or financial resources to participate. Emotions of shame or pride or anxiety felt by individuals are aspects of interacting with others. Social influence involving exhortation, directiveness or simple role modelling can alter the probability of a person becoming more or less active.

DOI: 10.4324/9781003025641-5

When we look to wider societal symbolism, sport is important not just in relation to individual health but also because it becomes part of a wider socio-political discourse of change. For example, here Nelson Mandela expressed the view that:

> Sport has the power to change the world. It has the power to inspire. It has the power to unite people in a way that little else does. It speaks to youth in a language they understand. Sport can create hope where once there was only despair. It is more powerful than government in breaking down racial barriers.
>
> (Mandela, speech at Laureas World Sports Awards, 25th May 2000)

Sport as a cultural phenomenon largely refers not only to active participation but also, to spectatorship. For every person who plays soccer there are thousands who sit and admire. Below this complexity will be explored using football and running as exemplars. We will also look at mobility in older and marginalised people.

The uneven participation in exercise

If we know that physical and mental health are improved by regular movement and exercise, then trends of such involvement in society are relevant to describe and account for. Before we address this point, a note will first be made about empirical evidence for the basic assumption that such activity is beneficial given the contemporary high rates of sedentary activity. Exercise brings some risks; in 'extreme sports' and any contact sports the more this is the case. However, overall the benefits of exercise are now well established and cannot be refuted. They are summarised in Box 5.1.

Box 5.1 Physical activity and health

- Physical activity is bodily movement resulting in energy expenditure – exercising, walking, gardening and doing housework. Regular physical activity is associated with reducing the risk of many illnesses and preventing rising rates of chronic conditions, having an impact earlier in the life course. Physical activity reduces mortality rates and improves quality of life with minimal or no safety concerns (Posadzki et al. 2020).
- Sedentary behaviour is waking behaviour with low energy expenditure – sitting/ reclining, watching TV, video gaming, using a computer. It is associated with: cancer, obesity, type 2 diabetes, cardiovascular diseases (CVD), stroke, hypertension, osteoarthritis,

lower back pain, depression, anxiety, dementia, chronic obstructive pulmonary disease (COPD), asthma, musculoskeletal conditions (Park et al. 2020).

- Walking, cycling, active recreation and participation in sport are associated with social and psychological benefits. They facilitate social inclusion, interactions with others, better learning and productivity in the workplace (Eime et al. 2013; Pereira et al. 2015).
- There is equivocal evidence for *specific* interventions seeking to increase inactivity amongst *targeted* groups (Corder et al. 2020).

Given the broad picture of the health benefits described in Box 5.1, the relationship the points make with inequality are relevant in two senses. First, is participation shaped by inequalities at source (such as locality or social group membership)? Second, are there consequential inequalities of participation, i.e., new forms, or the amplification of existing ones? With regard to the first question there is indeed evidence of unequal participation. That picture is summarised in Box 5.2.

Box 5.2 Examples of the physical inactivity gap

- There is consistent evidence of a higher prevalence of moderate–vigorous intensity physical activity in those at the top of the socio-economic scale compared with those at the bottom (Gidlow et al. 2006).
- Analysis of global physical activity data reveals the existence of worldwide activity inequality (Althoff et al. 2017).
- In higher-income countries there are greater inequality gaps between male and female activity levels, sport participation and attendance at sporting events (Cauwenberg et al. 2019).
- BME communities are more likely to be physically inactive. Women are more likely to be physically inactive than men, with the biggest gap between women and men found in South Asian people. In managerial and professional occupations those in the White British ethnic group were less likely to be physically inactive than most other ethnic groups (https://www.ethnicity-facts-figures.service.gov.uk/health/diet-and-exercise/physical-inactivity/latest).
- Sex differences in sporting participation are apparent, in most countries, women are less active than men (Althoff et al. 2017).
- Women's attitudes to physical activity in adulthood are shaped by childhood experiences of a lack of enjoyment and confidence in one's 'active' body. Stereotypical views about suitable candidates to participate in sport are likely to encourage insecurities around body image

and feeling constrained by cultural acceptability about being an active girl. Access to the built environment for exercise (e.g., safety, lighting) inhibit women from doing physical activity (The Lancet Public Health 2019).

Cultural distinctions, sport and exercise

The health benefits of moderate and vigorous physical activity are more evident in richer groups (Paudel et al. 2023). As is apparent from Box 5.2, the higher the social class one inhabits, the greater one's overall participation in sports and exercise. Involvement in sport, and regular exercise, have strong associations with education and social class (defined by occupation). In the UK there is less average leisure-time physical activity, and higher physical inactivity, amongst adults from lower, compared to higher socio-economic population groups. 'Not playing a sport' is accompanied by cultural practices, which include frequent TV watching, not reading books and not visiting art galleries. These trends are strongly associated with blue-collar work and unemployment (Bennett 2006). There is a constellation of habits here which confirms the pattern of distinctions and levels of cultural capital emphasised by Bourdieu (1979). He notes that dominant classes redefine the working classes' emphasis on physical strength as 'brute strength' (an 'unpredictable force of nature'), which compares unfavourably to the 'spiritual and intellectual strength' and 'self-control' they ascribe to themselves (p. 479). It is that second version of activity that marks out those who are not only more well-off but enjoy greater cultural capital. In turn, greater participation boosts social capital as well.

Those richest in cultural capital are least likely to be involved as participants in soccer with its working-class history (though increasingly they are spectators – see below). By contrast richer people tend to play their class-associated sports, such as rugby, polo, lacrosse and golf. Class distinction is evident in the participation in rugby football, with middle-class men predominating as both players and spectators.

That trend in relation to Rugby Union was reversed traditionally at the turn of the twentieth century though in relation to Rugby League. Originally, the latter split reflected the same 'gentleman and amateurs' division from lower-class players, who were paid as professionals, as in the game of cricket. Upper-class men played these sports as hobbies to demonstrate their masculine prowess, whilst those from poorer backgrounds were recruited using the cash nexus. The embodied power of masculine workers could be monetised in sport, whereas it was one of many pastimes for the better-off.

Exercise is commodified in a range of ways which impacts on who can do what. Sports equipment and gym provision in the 'fitness industry' is a contributor to GDP and employment globally. This industry and its products are sold unevenly: it is skewed towards those with the economic power to participate. The financial aspect of sporting participation is ever-present: the time and the equipment have a price attached. Skiing and horse riding follow an income gradient. The exclusivity of tennis and golf clubs structures this class division by the capacity to pay fees.

With these cost-inflected trends comes cultural features of etiquette and other aspects of social performativity. These are situations in which one's financial achievements and cultural know-how are both on display. Additionally, like life in the coffee shops in café society discussed previously, there are opportunities for accruing both social and cultural capital in interactions near to, but outside the sport itself, in the bars of club-houses. For these reasons, particular sports are often culturally off limits for poorer people: they cannot afford them and a lack of cultural capital keeps them at bay for reasons of both confidence and competence. Historically these exclusions have also been evident in relation to race and ethnicity (when membership discrimination resulted in Black and Jewish applicants being turned down in elite golf clubs in the USA).

There are wider implications of undertaking a highly valued culture or specific sports. These include the promotion and employment prospects for men at the expense of women. This point applies to the recruitment to elite-level jobs that historically have encouraged a cultural fit, in terms of participating in certain sports (e.g., rock climbing, lacrosse, sailing crew, squash, field hockey, tennis, scuba diving and marathon racing). These might be used at the point of recruitment as a 'story of self-actualization, growth, and drive', as a relevant basis for assessing job candidates, without reference to stated criteria of role suitability (Rivera 2015).

A matter of life and death: the revealing case of soccer

In the UK, football is conflated most of the time with soccer but middle-class people also call rugby, 'football'. With its first and commonest connotation, of soccer, the legendary Scottish manager of Liverpool FC, Bill Shankly, was asked about the importance of football in life. He famously replied:

> Some people believe football is a matter of life and death, I am very disappointed with that attitude. I can assure you it is much, much more important than that.

Notwithstanding this hyperbole, what is not in doubt is that globally soccer has become central to life, especially as a spectator sport, to many people in the population.

Health promoters view soccer as one amongst others that should be included as a *participatory* sport to enhance well-being, prevent morbidity and help recovery from illness. 'Football counts towards your recommended amount of aerobic activity' (https://www.nhsinform.scot/healthy-living/keeping-active/activities/football). Football understandably is incorporated into regimens for addressing physical inactivity, because of its combination of running, walking, sprinting and kicking. These can bring benefits including increased stamina, improvements to cardiovascular health, improved co-ordination as well increases in muscle and bone strength (https://www.nhsinform.scot/healthy-living/keeping-active/activities/football). However, to counter this salutogenic benefit, there is the caution that it is a contact sport, risking injury to the legs and the expectation to head the ball also brings the possibility of brain damage. (But rugby poses a greater danger to its participants (Frietag et al. 2015).)

Whilst the positive physiological effects of playing football are legitimately evidenced, the psychosocial aspects of the game are relevant as well. The middle-aged football supporter wearing their team's merchandise kit, who has never kicked a ball, constitutes part of the public health picture of the game. The feelings and symbolism associated with engaging with football have ramifications for living with class and social divisions. In an important sense it gives people the experience of entering a domain of freedom. The searching and finding of a site outside of the wretchedness and hassles of everyday life present an alternative reality. It is to use a term favoured by Cohen and Taylor (1975), an 'escape attempt' and, when successful, it affords positive emotions in people. Moreover, the social psychology of fandom potentially enhances a salutogenic effect.

Thus for health promoters to only, or mainly, discuss the link between football and well-being in terms of physiological efficiency is to offer a limited approach to the topic. Moreover, when we rise above this tendency of somatic reductionism, to explore the embedding social conditions of the game of football, their inequalities shape what is possible for individuals sharing the same societal exposure to the game. This is especially the case in relation to the pricing of tickets for elite games. A century ago live soccer was a low-price pastime as a spectator sport on a Saturday afternoon for working-class men and occasionally their children. Women were rarely seen in the crowd. Moreover, the inner lives of fans (whatever their social background) are relevant to consider. Mental health may be affected for good or bad in line with the recent success of a favoured team.

That inflexion of mental health is also mediated by social group membership: fans share an in-group allegiance and may project out their negative emotions onto competing teams and their supporters. At its worst this can culminate in a form of tribal violence. Thus fandom implicates the costs and benefits of tribalism (see the relevance of this in blue zones in Chapter 2). Sport spectatorship arouses the passions for good or bad and offers itself as both an escape attempt and form of existential ordering in the lives of fans. In this respect its comparison with religion is both obvious and pertinent. Its meaning to individual fans is exemplified here in this personal account:

> Well I feel I need to have something independent, something that is me and I can go away whenever I want to. I'm not sort of Dave, father, breadwinner, however you want to phrase it. Sometimes I'm the little lad down the street sort of ... It's mainly football, ... that has been consistent throughout my life and I think I need that sort of to stabilise me I think.
>
> (Rogers and Pilgrim 1997)

The socio-historical context of soccer

The current meaning of soccer to ordinary people has a relevant social history. Soccer originated as an elite game for Eton public schoolboys. However, it became popular primarily with the working class. Nineteenth-century mass migration to large cities for work as a result of industrialisation was accompanied by young men from the countryside with a passion for football. In England, a number of prominent clubs were formed as a result of groups of workers coming together, including Everton, Manchester United and Arsenal. Whilst the football pendulum, by the end of the twentieth century had rebalanced towards attracting a more middle-class audience, resulting from emergent commercialisation strategies, it has remained an essentially working-class game.

> Spectator behaviour at football matches has been seen as synonymous with groups of white working-class men – a form of organised working-class resistance which functions to 'reassert control in the face of the dominant middle classes'.
>
> (Waddington et al. 1989)

The customs, practices and ideas associated with football remain a strong part of working-class culture, despite an influx of newer middle-class interest in the fan base in recent decades. In particular across classes, it remains as a source of parochial pride. This positive link between class, culture and a socially valued healthy affirming product can be contrasted with the shame and disgust discussed about bodily expression of disadvantaged people as we discussed in Chapter 1.

'Sunderland till I die': the importance of locale

In the quote above from Bill Shankly, about football, life and death, he was making a generic existential point about the role of the game in modernity. There is a specific point as well to be made about localism. The Netflix series on the declining fortune of Sunderland FC is illuminative. The city is in the North East of England, like its nearby rival city (14 miles away), Newcastle, it thrived in the wake of the industrial revolution at the turn of the twentieth century with coal mining, steel making and shipbuilding. Both cities created well-known and successful clubs with a passionate (mainly) male proletarian fan base and this created a rivalrous relationship between the two places.

The symbolic role of football in that region emerged and became culturally poignant because of industrial precariousness. The first sign of this was in 1936, when 200 unemployed men from Jarrow, near Newcastle, marched to London to protest to the government about the closure of Palmer's shipyard. That acute crisis in British capitalism and the mass unemployment it witnessed returned in the 1980s. The North East like other areas of heavy industry in the UK suffered its material consequences of decline and raised levels of deprivation. Unemployment was high amongst the wreckage of a post-industrial rusting landscape.

That socio-economic context is the backdrop to the fate of clubs like Sunderland. If employment in the old industries had now disappeared, the cultural need for working-class solidarity (especially amongst men) remained. Tribal connection might retain a sense of camaraderie and joy, which used to be experienced in the past in the blue-collar workplace. If the locale of Sunderland was now objectively in a state of physical decline, then subjectively social and cultural capital might be re-animated with football fandom at its centre.

Sunderland Till I Die became popular for documenting this psychosocial transition, combining social history with personal accounts of the existential valorisation of football by ordinary people. The subjective ups and downs of the supporters at times mirrored the objective precariousness of the Sunderland locality. The club proudly in the elite of English football for so long, now suffered the ignominy of relegation from the Premier League. Accordingly, the accounts of fans are shot through with emotions of fear and desolation, countered at times by optimistic resistance. As this review of the series notes:

> Every goal, every mistake, every loss: they're all felt by more people than just the eleven men on the pitch and the several thousand crammed into the stands.
>
> (https://www.gq-magazine.co.uk/article/sunderland-til-i-die-netflix-review)

This interplay between the performance of a treasured team, and the mental health of its supporters, recurs in studies of football fandom. It reflects habitus in relation to our subjective rootedness in our class of origin. From another part of the country there is this account from an upwardly social mobile respondent:

> I view myself, as many of us do, as working class. As part of that, we have an in-built passion for football. Like millions before me, I would

> arrive home from school every day, get my kit on and play until it was pitch black.
>
> (https://www.watfordobserver.co.uk/sport/19714882.middle-class-politicians-keep-football/)

Watching football and being a fan (rather than playing) is a basis for feeling good and overcoming precariousness in everyday life and place and provides a means of 'fitting in'. In the past that normative function was highly gendered (football and being a boy went hand in glove). This began to change a little at the turn of this century, as the game began to accommodate young women, which fed through very recently into the rise of the professional women's game. The film *Bend It Like Beckham* reflected that shift. This also raised the matter of ethnicity. One of the actors was a British-born Asian, which pointed out an aspiration beyond gender (at present British-born African-Caribbean players are well-represented in the professional game, but this is not so much the case with those of South Asian heritage).

The more passive aspects of football participation may be linked to other inequalities early on in the life course, we noted earlier. Class differences in socialisation mean that the habitus of each is different. For example, one encourages soccer and in its commercial form this is a possible route for a few to fame and fortune for very talented working-class youngsters (once only boys but more recently girls as well).

By contrast rugby union in the countries it is played draws more from those with a richer background. As the latter has become more professionalised and robust it has become more dangerous, meaning that top-down commercial pressures are re-shaping the game at the time of writing (Scambler 2005). The latter author points out that the 'gentlemanly' etiquette of elite sports reflected a 'civilising process' (Elias 1978). With commercialisation, the game has begun to incorporate violent brute strength in the quest for success.

Sports participation was always high in a private school context and remained so. This can be contrasted in the UK with state schools losing playing fields. This has encouraged physical activity in the former version of habitus, which then converts into greater adult participation. As one recent study concluded, 'In effect, the mid- and upper-middle-class children were already sporting and cultural omnivores by the final years of primary schooling' (Wheeler et al. 2019, 89). These class distinctions have been added to by the distinction between male and female socialisation to which we now turn.

Masculinity and team sports

Whether we think of the 'playing fields of Eton' or the concrete playgrounds of state schools, boys have been afforded the opportunity to practice being a certain type of 'man'. Their heroes on the soccer, rugby or cricket field offered imagined possibilities and affiliations. As Swain (2000, 101) points out, 'by the time they have reached the age of 10 or 11, many of the boys will have spent thousands of hours, almost in rehearsal, of trying to look like, and emulate, their professional heroes'.

Masculinities which coalesce around the 'beautiful game' of soccer have been used in innovative health promotion, with some success. This has drawn upon the psychological dimension of male socialisation especially in working-class culture. Football Fans in Training (FFIT) was a novel way of using a passion for football to override traditional, more stigmatised ways of engaging with the risks to health (Gray et al. 2013).

FFIT works through accessing the value-identification about football, as a successful way of encouraging overweight men to attend weight management groups. By working with the enthusiasm and feelings that working-class male fans have about their football club the programme has shown effective results. FFIT gives access to behind-the-scene fans' 'home' professional clubs using these as highly valued environments for programmes of dietary advice and sessions of pitch-side physical activity. Participants valued the tribal connections of humour, camaraderie and peer support in order to encourage changes to everyday ways of living.

Masculinity and the influence on men's vision of themselves fed into their willingness to participate in healthy lifestyle programmes, when other traditional interventions had failed. The reasons for the success of this programme related to

> the creation of culturally bonded groups, through perceived commonalities and shared effervescent experience, and supportive discourses that challenged some potentially-damaging masculine orthodoxies allowed men not only to think differently, but also to support each other in making changes to their practices.
>
> (Bunn et al. 2018)

Whilst working-class men in considerable need of reducing their health risk might seemingly have benefitted from this use of hegemonic masculinity, on a broader level this may have been at the expense of women (despite recent efforts to increase the visibility of womens' soccer). Soccer in schools for girls is now being encouraged more and this upstream change is slowly being reflected in adult participation, including the professional game for women. There is an expanding culture of playing and appreciating football for both sexes – expressed in a 'new age' of media coverage (e.g., more coverage of the women's FIFA World Cup tournament and more female soccer commentators). However, there are also signs of a backlash to progress in sexual equality. There is still a culture of misogyny in which women are perceived, at times, as being sexual objects and are discounted more generally in the culture of fandom (Pope et al. 2022).

Turning to race, this has become a complex and at times controversial matter in the professional game. Historically, practices of institutional racism have limited minority access to senior organisational positions (Bradbury 2013). Black and ethnic minority players have suffered direct racism from fans at times. Occasionally this trend has been reflected on the pitch, with White players accused of racist slurs against competitors. In turn this has stimulated the growth of anti-racist campaigns from football associations. The anticipated risk of racism may be off-putting to both amateur and professional participants in soccer today. That risk also applies to Black and ethnic minority fans attending games as well (https://yougov.co.uk/topics/sport/articles-reports/2021/08/26/third-ethnic-minority-football-fans-have-experienc).

Thus when we start to unpick the social context of soccer in the past few decades it is a window into a range of psychosocial matters, including class variations in participation, White racism and hegemonic masculinity. We can distinguish between its relevance for well-being, when it is played, and when it is watched passively; this is not an either/or but a both/and matter. Certainly efforts at health promotion that only focus on its physiological benefits only tell half of the story.

Soccer had elite origins but it was soon proletarianised. This led to it being both a route for social mobility for young talented players, but more widely it became a focus for working-class tribalism in localities. The life and death discourse emerging from these economically determined processes was noted and resonated with other versions of tribalism or even national loyalties in wider society. We also need to take into account how this wider picture was modified by the end of the twentieth century by consideration of sex and ethnicity.

The aesthetics of running

Like football, running is presented in public health terms, as a fairly simple activity of aerobic exercise, fending off the risk to health of being excessively sedentary. Recreational running is viewed pragmatically as a cheap (no expensive gym membership) and accessible form of exercise, made possible in a range of environments. It is potentially suited to everyone, given the requirement for little expertise, experience or specialist equipment and the ease with which it can be fitted into everyday lives for those pressed for time. Running is seemingly a panacea for addressing inequalities. However, this unproblematic view of running hides an underlying promotion of 'an embodiment of middle-classness that naturalizes gender and age inequalities whilst also individualising responsibility for them' (Abbas 2004, 159). In other words, social inequalities are backgrounded, whereas individual agency about improving health is valorised.

Running has the advantage to its promoters, and the appeal to its participants, of us controlling the health of our bodies using a particular version of physical discipline. This brings with it, emotional release and sensations of comfort, as well as the psychological benefits of identity building and improved self-worth.

It might even represent for poorer people an escape attempt (Cohen and Taylor 1992) as depicted in the classic novel *The Loneliness of the Long-Distance Runner* from 1959. In this story, running provides an emotional and physical way out of miserable life circumstances. It refers to a teenager from a bleak working-class area and home with dismal life prospects, who takes up long-distance running as an antidote to social alienation. He deliberately fails to cross the line, though in the lead, as a show of independence and rebellion against his incarceration in borstal.

Running in this fictional account acted as a form of reflection and response to becoming aware of the class divisions in 1950s Britain. This captures the potential of running as a force for personal liberation and autonomy. However, in terms of contemporary class narratives running is more (though by no means exclusively) a sport of the affluent and the well-educated. Here is an account reflecting this class inflexion:

> Now that I am a full-time mom and part-time writer, my schedule isn't particularly easy – but it does afford me flexibility. I am not solely burdened by concerns of making ends meet, thanks to my husband's career. I also live in an area where generally safe, runnable trails are nearly as common as roads. This is where my 'commitment to exercise' and inherent privilege as an upper-middle-class woman have an inextricable link.
> (https://medium.com/the-establishment/the-remarkable-privilege-of-running-785ab4e9375c)

Running creates personal and idiosyncratic feelings and meanings. Recreational running can foster a form of appreciation, which is wedded to a set of values and class-aligned capital. It happens alone or in communities but is in common with football above, constituted via shared identities and subcultures. Distinctions are made, for example, between athletes, runners and joggers. Runners quietly get to know their place, whether or not that becomes explicit in conversation with others.

The aesthetic and pleasurable experience of habitual long-term running in open and beautiful landscapes (such as the Lake District) generates, what Nettleton (2013 and 2015) refers to as, 'existential capital'. This is an embodied gratification that serves as an attractor that binds those who appreciate 'feelings of being alive with, and in, the fells'. 'Sporting capital', more generally refers to a shared set of specific performance goals and training techniques, amongst groups of veteran runners (Hitchings and Latham 2017).

This embodiment has a range of aspects, which include the experience of, and conversations about, particular running environments. These might be exciting or boring. Other experiential considerations include the quality of air at different points, encounters with dogs and other obstacles and threats as well as the forbearance at times about the loneliness of running. The loneliness of the long-distance runner is multifaceted.

Running environments and social class

This sense of being alive, via regular bouts of running, might be less readily available to those who have less conducive environments to run in and this will be an impediment to doing this at all. The running 'for all' strategy, from health promoters, ignores ways in which running plays out differentially for people in different social circumstances.

The pleasure associated with running is established through movement and sensation (e.g., the rhythm), through contact with and use of technologies and of everyday routine. Ideally people might run unencumbered in a wide open space, whereas subjectively other spaces might be exciting or stressful. A commuter-runner with a rucksack on their back may feel energised or irritated by his or her challenge. Running with a bag as a commuter is 'an encumbrance that mediates and transforms the embodied experiences of run-commuting in a multitude of ways' (Cook and Larsen 2022).

Some outdoor runners are attracted and motivated by the fact their run takes them out into the hustle and bustle of everyday life in their locality, whereas others only want greenery. If they have the choice, runners learn to blend in seamlessly with their preferred routes. This interaction between the runner and their places of running makes them even part of the 'weather landscape', speeding or plodding through the cold and rain, or avoiding it at the outset with the benefit of a local forecast.

Whilst these agentic aspects of running are important for any runner, the options for some are more varied than others. For example, immediate access from the home to green spaces (or via a short car ride away) is an option for some but not others. Those car-less in a congested and polluted poor urban environment are obliged to accept it, or abandon the effort as unwelcoming. Compare that scenario to the fell runner, noted above, or those enjoying more spacious city areas. Another distinction to bear in mind, other than access to preferred running spaces is the use and existential preference for devices, which we turn to next.

The psychosocial aspects of exercise devices

The optimisation, via personal choices, of the running experience (and exercise more generally) can now be attained using new digital technology. This is both a matter of affordability (those who have less money have difficulties prioritising this, in any exercise they partake in) and of performativity, as superiority in exercise can be displayed by possessing 'the best' aids and apps. The latter is an extension from previous times of wearing the best clothes for the task. Clothes were fit for a purpose (in relation to wind resistance and temperature regulation), but now potentially electronic devices can take the runner onto a new level of efficiency and personal performance.

Success in events or personal performance can be monitored and displayed, using specialised equipment and technology (Qviström 2013). If this has been associated with elite competitive events, it has also been extended to its individualised use on the one hand, and connections with those with a similar lifestyle, on the other. We see this around us in developed countries in which runners publicly are wearing sports watches/wearable devices and their viewing of specialist apps, on their smartphones. Running with visible technology is a social performance.

These devices signal access to, and attainment of, a type of esoteric knowledge, especially about the body. The display on the equipment then also affords a social display, as well as being a basic physiological measure of attainment and improvement. 'My personal best' becomes both an inner driver and a boast or confession to others. The runner with the specialised electronic technology indicates an improved form of self-possession, aligned with middle-class habitus of being in control of their health and fate. Moreover, the precision afforded by such devices signals that the owner has higher levels of knowledge about how running *should be done* implying a moral discourse. We see here then how new technology has afforded new forms of distinction between the haves and the have-nots, the worthy and the unworthy, the talented and the ordinary, those in the know and those not, about an activity, which is seemingly so natural, simple and available to all in society. Available 'yes' but simple 'no', because of the many psychosocial cross-currents, which define and afford it. (An elephant in the room here is that some people are physically unable to run at all.)

The distinction between the more and less affluent runner, afforded by expensive devices, has been confirmed empirically. Individuals from affluent social milieus are more likely to use exercise-related apps and to participate in online social networks. Those from lower social class backgrounds show greater hesitancy and reluctance to use physical activity digital devices or to participate in self-quantification (Larsson and Larsson 2021).

Another consideration when explaining this distinction (apart from cost) is confidence in surveillance systems. Disadvantaged people tend to lack trust in the latter more often, (though clearly there are individual differences in suspiciousness within all classes). A reinforcing point, beyond trends in resistance to surveillance, is the experienced *futility* of self-surveillance. Poorer people have less confidence in personal control, which is a theme that repeats in other chapters in this book. What is the point in looking at personal data if one is personally fatalistic about health?

This matter of locus of control is then class inflected. Richer and more educated people tend to believe more strongly in the prospect or actuality of self-control about their morbidity and mortality. Their fate is more likely to be seen to be in their own hands, which encourages forms of restraint and self-discipline, with self-monitoring, using technology, recently playing a reinforcing role in this regard. An analogy here is self-monitoring in relation to dietary content, which we discussed in Chapter 3. Exercise and diet are the two mainstays of health self-promotion.

With that class-inflected habitus about health self-promotion in mind, the public display of digital health technology mediates a recurring message about self-control and the celebration of worthy independent effort in life. This subtly confirms not just moral worthiness but the runner's social status, relative to others. Salient individual *independence* marks them out. Whether or not that is the conscious intention of individual runners, it is certainly one of the micro-social consequences.

By contrast the habitus of poorer people is characterised more by *interdependence*. The non-use of technology (as with a relative indifference to sports attire) creates a shared acceptance of running in the particular ways of poorer environments. The 'value-added' concern with not just the running, but also how it is clothed and technologically elaborated, displays to the world a different way of being a healthy adult in richer runners. 'Expressive independence', is more typical of those from situations of affluence, who have fewer routine worries about making ends meet and getting through the challenges of life. This affords an opportunity to display, not just enact, their personal interests and achievements for public appreciation.

Apart from this display of distinction function, devices also modulate ways of thinking. There is a motivational dimension to their use. Promoted as consumer durables, with engaged recipients, they are incorporated into regimes of thinking and experience and now form an expansive and expanding market of watches, GPS devices, Heart Rate Monitors (HRMs), specialist trainers and clothing. These have become part of the semiotic package of being a good runner, even when this applies to recreation, not competition (McCormack et al. 2013).

Knowledge and discussion about the nuanced pros and cons of devices feed into status solidarity and class distinctions. The unique selling points of particular devices meld with the unique status of this particular runner and their particular class-related peers. Savvy, and digitally aware and informed participants, tend to be hyper-aware of advertising and promotional methods, which are used to engage consumers. Thus being a *discerning and critical* consumer of devices legitimises the importance of them in principle.

This is not about consumer resistance but consumer discernment, which contributes to market competition. If that is the commercial implication, then interpersonally this also leads to status comparisons. Social comparisons will always favour those already at an advantage, compared to poorer citizens. Social defeat in the poor will then trigger demoralisation and a withdrawal into passivity, when and if these social comparisons are experienced in practice in shared settings.

A countervailing trend to disrupt these patterns of distinction and unfavourable social comparisons are interventions to encourage 'low tech' collective activation, which we now consider.

Collectivised sport and parkrun

The organisation of running spaces range from those that are organised to those which are more disparate and ad hoc. They include joggers at lunchtime or directly from domestic settings, as well as running for exercise and fitness and the multiplicity of organised events, such as marathons, charity runs and local running clubs (Janssen et al. 2017). In these varying situations, individuals express their body capital. This is like Nettleton's (2013) fell runners, who did not do extra exercises or think about reaching an idealised body image as their goal. Instead they were maximising their enjoyment by keeping their body in an active state and experiencing movement. This was about an existential process, not a measurable goal to be recorded and witnessed by others in a state of appreciation.

This body capital can also deepen an engagement with running, other runners and club activities. The *Parkrun* is another running arena, which offers a space for 'collective bodywork' and sociability, whereby participants simultaneously enact and experience a sense of being 'all in this together'. *Parkrun* is a charity operating on a global basis organising free, weekly five kilometres outdoor events in the community, for people of all ages. It encourages runners, walkers or volunteers and is designed to be attractive to those who might not have thought about running before. Those using the runs regularly experience increases in weekly physical activity levels, report improved fitness, weight control and mental well-being (Stevinson et al. 2015).

Parkrun seemingly has a very strong pull. It is seen as a novel social movement and public health intervention. Like the football fan's zeal it carries a sense of religious conviction, driven by feelings of well-being achieved and experienced individually and shared collectively as 'life changing' (Jones 2021). Like football fans in training discussed above, the collective elements of *Parkrun* seem to mitigate certain individualising effects of health responsibilisation. Instead it draws upon a sense of reciprocity and being part of a community. It potentially acts as a forum for diminishing inequities associated with the practice of running.

Parkrun provides new participants with the means to negotiate the potential perceived risks in starting to run in a way, that reconciles feelings and experiences of being an 'unfit-runner'. This initiative like that of the overweight football fans training at their preferred club brings together not just those who are amateur but those who are not the usual candidates for fitness regimes. This generates collective efficacy and raises the game for individual participants, many of whom have the paradoxical starting point of lacking fitness or being impaired in their functioning.

Despite the open wide and visible spaces within which *Parkrun* takes place on a weekly basis, and those who are from less advantaged backgrounds benefiting once they have become a Parkrunner, one failing point is related to access and participation. *Parkrun* does not seem to attract significantly from more deprived areas and areas with higher ethnic minority, which are the very places from which health benefits could accrue. This reminds us again of the incorrigible persistence of social inequalities that we noted in Chapter 1 (Smith et al. 2019).

Mobility is not always exercise

Being on the move, whether through exercise or seated transport, is relevant to health and well-being. It is socially patterned and it changes over the life course. Car use comes with health and environmental costs, but for deprived populations it promotes psycho-social well-being. Car ownership confers social status; this is true across the class gradient. It is a key cognitive resource in bridging the gap between an individual's desires and their particular circumstance. Moreover, in a car-dependent era with a lack of comprehensive other options, travel without a car can often be difficult and inconvenient, particularly for vulnerable groups including older people (Goodman et al. 2012).

Putting aside the physiological benefits of exercise, which are negated by car use, getting around by any means is still the basis for social contact and can give meaning to people in everyday life. Getting out and doing things brings with it the opportunities for both of these human needs. Such activity fills time, and it staves off boredom. Without it, people are more likely to report poor health and limited participation in social activities.

Mobility inequality is defined as disadvantages produced by unequal access to resources for physical accessibility (Ferreira et al. 2012). This means poor access to desired destinations, such as shops, leisure activities, homes of friends and health care. Unequal access to these resources, leads to restricted daily movement. People with disabilities and older adults experience the most limited mobility, reducing their social contact and their access to sporting and leisure activities. Mobility, rather than exercise per se, is the vehicle not only to maintain social contact but also for retention of cognitive skills and a sense of citizenship. Accordingly, independence, a sense of well-being and social engagement all are reliant on mobility and so they are jeopardised when movement is not enabled for vulnerable and disadvantaged groups (Meijering 2021).

These slower and less-challenging expectations of mobility still bring with them a number of impediments and enablers, such as the weather and the physical state of routes. For those able to walk but not run, pavements may have trip hazards and their state of repair is inflected by how rich or poor the neighbourhood is. The availability of resting points, with benches, may shape a person's confidence to walk out. Busy roads with few crossing points can induce fear in those who are frail and this may inhibit them from venturing out. This point is more salient in relation to wheelchair users or those with sight impairments. In the latter regard, note how some pedestrian light crossings have no sound indicator.

The totality of all enabling or disabling environmental factors has been conceptualised as 'infrastructure capital'. This refers to the opportunity to move, which is shaped by public service provision, the maintenance of the local built environment, and the direct financial costs of travel (Musselwhite and Scott 2019). As with the case of running, this is a reminder that what seems like direct and democratically available free form of movement (i.e., getting out of one's home as a road passenger, or walking in one's immediate neighbourhood) is actually constrained by a complex web of extrinsic factors. Accordingly, this becomes a scenario of movement inequality.

Conclusions

This chapter began by noting the traditional support of health promoters for physical exercise in the population. It went on to explore the psycho-social implications of this basic advice and an understanding of the fine-grain differences in the social context of people trying to keep healthy by exercising. This situated approach reveals complexity in a range of ways related to financial means, locale, sex, ethnicity and age. It also draws attention to the variegated existential implications in a population; we imbue exercise with meanings and it is a vehicle for social and cultural capital. It indicates our place in society and affords our experience of status within it. The macro version reminds us that sport and exercise are commodified and marketised.

The duality of this picture is most obvious in relation to understanding the complexity of spectatorship. The main example was of football fandom in post-industrial settings in the UK. Finally we noted that mobility and exercise are linked but not the same. The importance for disabled or elderly people to get out and about implicates a range of subjective needs (from cognitive skills to citizenship) and objective constraints. The latter includes access to transport and the physical safety of the built environments.

References

Abbas, A. 2004. "The Embodiment of Class, Gender and Age Through Leisure: A Realist Analysis of Long Distance Running." *Leisure Studies* 23 (2): 159–175.

Althoff, T., R. Sosič, J.L. Hicks, A.C. King, S.L. Delp, and J. Leskovec. 2017. "Large-Scale Physical Activity Data Reveal Worldwide Activity Inequality." *Nature* 547 (7663): 336–339. doi: 10.1038/nature23018. Epub 2017 Jul 10.

Bennett, T. 2006. "Distinction on the Box: Cultural Capital and the Social Space of Broadcasting." *Cultural Trends* 15 (2–3): 193–212.

Bourdieu, P. 1979. *Distinction: A Social Critique of the Judgement of Taste*, trans. Richard Nice. Cambridge, MA: Harvard University Press.

Bradbury, S. 2013. "Institutional Racism, Whiteness and the Under-Representation of Minorities in Leadership Positions in Football in Europe." *Soccer & Society* 14 (3): 296–314.

Brooke, S. 2001. "Gender and Working Class Identity in Britain During the 1950s." *Journal of Social History* 34 (4): 773–795.

Bunn, C., C. Donnachie, S. Wyke, et al. 2018. "Can Professional Football Clubs Deliver a Weight Management Programme for Women: A Feasibility Study." *BMC Public Health* 18: 1330.

Cauwenberg, V., J. De Clerq, B. Deforche, et al. 2019. "Accuracy and Inequalities in Physical Activity Research." *The Lancet Global Health* 7 (2): 183–184.

Cohen, S., and L. Taylor. 1992. *Escape Attempts: The Theory and Practice of Resistance in Everyday Life*, 2nd edn, 262. Abingdon Oxford: Routledge.

Cook, S., and J. Larsen. 2022. "Geographies of Running Cultures and Practices." *Geography Compass* 16 (10): 1–13.

Corder, K., S.J. Sharp, S.T. Jong, et al. 2020. "Effectiveness and Cost-Effectiveness of the Goactive Intervention to Increase Physical Activity Among UK Adolescents: A Cluster Randomised Controlled Trial." *PLoS Medicine* 17 (7): e1003210.

Elias, N. 1978. "*The Civilising Process*. Oxford: Blackwell.

Eime, R., J. Young, Harvey, et al. 2013. "A Systematic Review of the Psychological and Social Benefits of Participation in Sport for Children and Adolescents: Information Development of a Conceptual Model of Health Through Sport." *International Journal of Behavioral Nutrition and Physical Activity* 10 (1): 1–21.

Freitag, A., G. Kirkwood, S. Scharer, R. Ofori-Asenso, and A.M. Pollock. 2015. "Systematic Review of Rugby Injuries in Children and Adolescents Under 21 Years." *British Journal of Sports Medicine* 49 (8): 511–519.

Gidlow, C., L. Johnson, D. Corne, N. Ellis, and D. James. 2006. "A Systematic Review of the Relationship Between Socio-Economic Position and Physical Activity." *Health Education Journal* 65 (4): 338–367.

Goodman, A., C. Guell, J. Panter, N.R. Jones, and D. Ogilvie. 2012. "Healthy Travel and the Socio-Economic Structure of Car Commuting in Cambridge, UK: A Mixed-Methods Analysis." *Social Science & Medicine* 74 (12): 1929–1938.

Gray, C.M., K. Hunt, N. Mutrie, et al. 2013. "Football Fans in Training: The Development and Optimization of an Intervention Delivered Through Professional Sports Clubs to Help Men Lose Weight, Become More Active and Adopt Healthier Eating Habits." *BMC Public Health* 13: 232.

Hitchings, R., and A. Latham. 2017. "How 'Social' Is Recreational Running? Findings from a Qualitative Study in London and Implications for Public Health Promotion." *Health & Place* 46: 337–343. doi: 10.1016/j.healthplace.2016.10.003. Epub 2016 Dec 18.

Janssen, I., K.C. Roberts, and W. Thompson. 2017. "Compliance by Canadians Aged 10 to 17 Years with the Canadian Guidelines of 24-Hour Movement for Children and Youth." *Health Promotion and Chronic Disease Prevention in Canada: Research, Policy and Practice* 37 (11): 413–420.

Jones, E. 2021. *How Parkrun Changed Our Lives*. Hebden Bridge: Gristone.

Larsson, H., and B. Larsson. 2021. "Social Stratification of Physical Activity: An Exploration Into How Logics of Practice Affect Participation in Movement Culture." *Physical Education and Sport Pedagogy* 28 (3): 213–228.

McCormack, B., J. Rycroft-Malone, K. DeCorby, et al. 2013. "A Realist Review of Interventions and Strategies to Promote Evidence-Informed Healthcare: A Focus on Change Agency." *Implementation Science* 8: 107. doi: 10.1186/1748-5908-8-107.

Meijering, L. 2021. "Towards Meaningful Mobility: A Research Agenda for Movement Within and Between Places in Later Life." *Ageing & Society* 41: 711–723.

Musselwhite, C., and T. Scott. 2019. "Developing a Model of Mobility Capital for an Ageing Population." *International Journal of Environmental Research and Public Health* 16 (18): 3327.

Nettleton, S. 2013. "Cementing Relations Within a Sporting Field: Fell Running in the English Lake District and the Acquisition of Existential Capital." *Cultural Sociology* 7: 196–210.

Nettleton, S. 2015. "Fell Runners and Walking Walls: Towards a Sociology of Living Landscapes and Aesthetic Atmospheres as an Alternative to a Lakeland Picturesque." *British Journal of Sociology* 66 (4): 759–778.

Park, J.H., J.H. Moon, H.J. Kim, M.H. Kong, and Y.H. Oh. 2020. "Sedentary Lifestyle: Overview of Updated Evidence of Potential Health Risks." *Korean Journal of Family Medicine* 41 (6): 365–373. doi: 10.4082/kjfm.20.0165. Epub Nov 19.

Paudel, S., M. Ahmadi, P. Phongsavan, M. Hamer, and E. Stamatakis. 2023. "Do Associations of Physical Activity and Sedentary Behaviour with Cardiovascular Disease and Mortality Differ Across Socioeconomic Groups? A Prospective Analysis of Device-Measured and Self-Reported UK Biobank Data." *British Journal of Sports Medicine* 8: bjsports-2022-105435.

Pereira, M., B. Coombes, T. Comans, et al. 2015. "The Impact of Onsite Work Place Health-Enhancing Activity Interventions on Worker Productivity: A Systematic Review." *Occupational and Environmental Medicine* 72 (6): 401–412.

Pope, S., and W.J Cleland, et al. 2022. "Men's Football Fandom and the Performance of Progressive and Misogynistic Masculinities in a New Age' of UK Women's Sport (2022)." *Sociology* 56 (4): 730–748.

Posadzki, P., D. Pieper, R. Bajpai, et al. 2020. "Exercise/Physical Activity and Health Outcomes: An Overview of Cochrane Systematic Reviews." *BMC Public Health* 20: 1724.

Qviström, M. 2013. "Landscapes with a Heartbeat: Tracing a Portable Landscape for Jogging in Sweden (1958–1971)." *Environment and Planning* 45 (2): 312–328.

Rivera, L.A. 2015. "Go with Your Gut: Emotion and Evaluation in Job Interviews." *American Journal of Sociology* 120 (5): 1339–1389. doi: 10.1086/681214.

Rogers, A., and D. Pilgrim. 1997. "The Contribution of Lay Knowledge to the Understanding and Promotion of Mental Health." *Journal of Mental Health* 6 (1): 23–36.

Scambler, G. 2005. *Sport Society: History Power and Culture*, 211. Milton Keynes Buckinghamshire: Mc Graw-Hill Education.

Smith, R.A., P.P. Schneider, R. Cosulich, et al. 2021. "Socioeconomic Inequalities in Distance to and Participation in a Community-Based Running and Walking Activity: A Longitudinal Ecological Study of Parkrun 2010 to 2019." *Health & Place* 71: 102626. ISSN 1353-8292.

Smith, R., R. Spaaij, and B. McDonald. 2019. "Migrant Integration and Cultural Capital in the Context of Sport and Physical Activity: A Systematic Review." *International Migration & Integration* 20: 851–868.

Stevinson, C., G. Wiltshire, and M. Hickson. 2015. "Facilitating Participation in Health-Enhancing Physical Activity: A Qualitative Study of Parkrun." *International Journal of Behavioural Medicine* 22: 170–177.

Swain, J. 2000. "The Moneys Good, the Fame's Good, the Girls Are Good; the Role of Play Ground Football in the Construction of Young Boys Masculinity in Junior School." *British Journal of Sociology of Education* 21 (1): 97–106.

The Lancet Public Health. 2019. "Time to Tackle the Physical Activity Gender Gap." *Lancet Public Health* 4 (8): e360.

Waddington, D., K. Jones, and C. Critcher. 1989. *Flashpoints: Studies in Disorder*. Abingdon Oxford: Routledge.

Wankel, L.M., and B.G. Berger. 1990. "The Psychological and Social Benefits of Sport and Physical Activity." *Journal of Leisure Research* 22 (2): 167–182.

Wheeler, S., K. Green, M. Thurston, et al. 2019. "Social Class and the Emergent Organised Sporting Habits of Primary-Aged Children." *European Physical Education Review* 25 (1): 89–108.

Wilmot, E.G., C.L. Edwardson, F.A. Achana, et al. 2012. "Sedentary Time in Adults and the Association with Diabetes, Cardiovascular Disease and Death: Systematic Review and Meta-Analysis." *Diabetologia* 55: 2895–2905.

6 Ordinary distress and loneliness

Introduction

Loneliness constitutes an unwanted subjective state that stems from the 'perceived discrepancy between desired and actual social relationships' (McKenna-Plumley et al. 2020), a lack of social intimacy and a deficiency in social relationships (Weiss 1973). It is a socially patterned state, unequally distributed, with greater prevalence amongst younger and older people, migrants, those with long-term conditions and ethnic minority groups (Lasgaard et al. 2016; Salway et al. 2020).

Loneliness has been framed at times as a significant public health problem or even emergency or 'epidemic'. It is a predictor of both poor mental and physical health status and *vice versa*. Chronic loneliness increases mortality by 26%, with claims that it has a similar risk equivalence to that of smoking 100 cigarettes per day (Holt-Lunstad et al. 2015). The concept is useful in thinking about health in biopsychosocial terms. Metaphysically it invites other ways of reflecting on a recurring social–existential state, which is relevant to how we live with loneliness in our daily lives.

Social isolation has been understood traditionally in both existential and social–scientific terms. These different starting points, one highly subjective and the other examining external social processes, have complemented one another. Søren Kierkegaard one of the founders of modern existentialism talked of our lonely angst-ridden state of 'sickness unto death' (Grøn 2008). Sigmund Freud explored the psychopathology of everyday life and our constant state of anxiety, to be either expressed (our personal version of neurosis) or fended off (our personal forms of distorting defence mechanisms). He also examined the relationship between mourning and melancholia (Freud 1917).

These recurring inner states emerge in an interpersonal context, and so they need to be considered in terms of not just being on 'our own', but being with others as well. At times, the tension or gap between aloneness and relationships with others (desired or avoided) can become part of the recurrent picture of anxiety, sadness and loneliness. That tension between solitude and relationality is played out differently over time. All people have a capacity for experiencing loneliness, but this always happens in *this* person in their

DOI: 10.4324/9781003025641-6

particular life. And because of a shared unequal society that particularity bears exploration case by case and in terms of trends of loneliness in different social groups.

This chapter considers the naming and framing of distress and loneliness. We then move to the lonely citizen of capitalism, and the recurring importance of social networks in promoting and understanding the health of individuals.

Understanding the experience of distress and loneliness

Being part of a social species, and its interdependent character, humans have the recurring dilemma of balancing being alone and being with others. Within this recurring dilemma solitude and loneliness can be distinguished. Loneliness is a distressed subjective experience but solitude is characterised by calmness, enjoyment or even extraordinary spirituality in practice.

The psychoanalyst Donald Winnicott drew a useful distinction between the capacity to be alone and the compulsion to be alone (Winnicott 1965). The first represented a form of psychological maturity, whereas the second might indicate 'schizoid' withdrawal, depression or profound social anxiety. Thus a conceptual difference is that solitude is desirable but loneliness is not. Solitude is the choice to be alone and use that time either for reflection or simply enjoyment in one's own company. It is about being present with one's own self rather than the lack of companionship from others.

Being solitary has been a primary goal of hermits, pilgrims and religious itinerants. Across time and space they recur as positive role models, notably separating themselves from the daily norms of social interaction. They have demonstrated the potential benefits of contemplative solitude. In antiquity there was ambiguity about the lonesome traveller, as they might also be thought of as mad, but if they were calm then a spiritual quest might also be assumed (Rosen 1968).

Even here there are clear social divisions in the domestic arrangements for the enactment of solitude. Religious individuals of early Christendom lived on their own in solitude to escape the temptations of the world in hermitages, caves or rudimentary small buildings, located in deserts, mountains or forests. However, in the nineteenth century, some aristocrats built hermitages as places of retreat designed as an architectural feature in lavish grounds, which 'draw the eye' to the surrounding landscape for contemplation. Nevertheless in both cases the difference between solitude, as an actively chosen state, compared to loneliness remained. Today artists may opt to be alone in a state of unchecked imagination or creative melancholy. In a modified form the retreat, secular or religious, resonates with these positive features of solitude; so too with the writer's room, or the musician's or painter's studio.

When it comes to loneliness, loss and separation from others typically leads to distress and this is manifest across other animal species. We can all spot a trembling and whimpering dog tied to a post outside of a shop, waiting anxiously for its owner to return. Horses mourn a lost part of the herd or a stillborn foal, showing a sort of agitated depression, similar to human experiences. It is not surprising then that the empirical case made by the psychoanalyst John Bowlby, when developing his attachment theory, drew upon cross-species comparisons from ethology (the study of animals in their natural environment).

Thus the experience of 'loneliness' is not a single state but more of a constellation of reactions and emotions, composed of a wide variety of embodied responses that include fear, anger, resentment and sorrow. Most prominent is social anxiety; anxiety and loneliness can be viewed as overlapping states. For lonely people, this might be about social threat, which drives those fearing others to retreat from contact. Being alone may also lead to a lack of practice and confidence in being with others, creating a vicious circle of lonely avoidance. (In formal psychiatric terms, when social anxiety becomes chronic, it can invoke the diagnosis of 'avoidant personality disorder'.) In social terms, extreme shyness is framed as a medical disability. But however it is labelled, some people do find themselves dislocated from others in a distressed state.

If anxiety is commonly reported by lonely people, then so is depression. The very common co-presence of anxiety and depression in patients presenting in primary care with 'common mental disorders', has meant arguments for their acceptance as a unitary state (Tyrer 2022). Neither loneliness nor notions of 'clinical depression' are conceptually neat categories. They overlap with ordinary feelings of sadness, grumpy pessimism and a lack of motivation in daily life, as well as responses to clearly definable losses, such as mourning after death or divorce. Sadness is part of the human condition, and like anxiety can be claimed fairly as a natural given. Thus when loneliness is explored conceptually, arguably it has both pathological and very ordinary features.

Whereas depression is presumed to mean one *isolates* oneself from others, loneliness usually assumes a *lack of interaction* with others, and feeling alienated from them. Loneliness then might be distinguished from depression, because it reflects the discrepancy between actual and desired social relationships or a deficit between the actual and expected number and quality of social relations and interactions. Depression is a common form of distress attending a wide variety of circumstances, not just loneliness.

Once relationality is considered as the bridge between the individual and society, then this micro-sociological focus can invoke Durkheim's notion of 'anomie' and Marx's of 'alienation'. That consideration responds to the request of C.W. Mills to exercise a 'sociological imagination' and his suggestion that it is possible to trace the links between 'private troubles' and 'public issues' (Mills 1959). In the case of loneliness, the latter involves diverse elements, including economic and social success or its lack, divorce, children leaving home, job loss, low-status employment, alcohol pricing, transport policies, street crime and, simply, urbanicity. Together these increase the risk of social marginality and, within that trend, some individuals will be more vulnerable to withdrawal or social exclusion than others. Loneliness reflects contingent norms of civic participation and social cohesion, and the vulnerability of these in the young and old is important to note (Schirmer and Michailakis 2016). We return to this point about the life span in Chapter 8. Some patterns of loneliness are summarised in Box 6.1.

Box 6.1 Private troubles and public issues: the social patterning of loneliness

Disadvantaged socio-economic position is linked with loneliness, so too with those who are widowed (Kearns et al. 2015; Eckard 2018). The most vulnerable to loneliness are younger men living in individualistic cultures. Loneliness decreases with age and is greater in men than in women (Childs and Lawton 2019). Divorced men report higher levels of loneliness compared to women. For older people, the risk of loneliness is highest in the least wealthy groups and lowest in the wealthiest (Bosma et al. 2015). The predisposition to loneliness is also mediated and compounded through having a chronic illness. In turn, the risk of the latter is highest in those who are poorest. For those with a long-term condition, there is a high association, with loneliness impacting on previous roles and ability to stay connected to previously valued roles and opportunities for social participation (Vassilev et al. 2014).

The discussion of loneliness recently has often been in the context of mental health challenges. This entails it being considered in an overlapping way with depression (as a 'common mental disorder' in routine life) but also with Post-Traumatic Stress Disorder (PTSD). The latter is diagnosed in the wake of demonstrable 'nervous shocks' to people. These might include personal assaults, warfare, terror attacks, natural disasters and outbreaks of diseases. Traumatised people sometimes are wary of others and they seek the protection of individual isolation, which can then trigger long-term social dislocation.

This blurring of the boundaries between concepts reminds us that while human distress (basically sadness and anxiety) is broadly a natural given, and even demonstrable in other species, how it is understood, experienced and shaped is dependent upon fine-grain differences in social life. As with loneliness, anxiety and depression can be considered common mental health problems or variations in human experience characterised by distress.

The lonely citizen of capitalism

The relationship between social contexts, in which distress and loneliness become salient is important to consider. Historically, loneliness, as a state of sadness and angst, was associated particularly with the early nineteenth century. During that post-Enlightenment period, and the emergence of modernity and an increasingly industrialised and urban mode of living in the West, loneliness emerged as an important existential consideration.

Before 1800, the English word 'loneliness' was scarce, because it had no reference point, in the external realities of everyday life for ordinary people. Rather, social arrangements with people living in small close groups, relatively physically isolated but governed by notions of the local community as a common good, as well as a belief in God, meant people never felt truly alone, or if they did it was not apparent in the discourse of the period (Alberti 2019). By the mid-twentieth century, loneliness and the capacity to be alone, without distress, attracted the interests of psychoanalysts, as Donald Winnicott noted earlier. Writing in a period of social and economic adjustment after the Second World War, with lost lives and children displaced from their relatives, temporarily or permanently, Winnicott, like his psychoanalytical colleague John Bowlby, focused upon the type and quantity of attachments shaping our mental health, especially in the everyday life of the family (Winnicott 1957).

This post-war period in Europe and North America invited a bridging form of understanding, between the subjective and the objective in psychoanalytical reasoning: relationality as both an external context and an internalised part of our inner lives (confusingly called 'object relations' by analysts even though the allusion was to people). Viewing loneliness in this relational way points up specific biographical contexts from both the past (what has happened to people in their particular childhood or as adults experiencing trauma or loss) and the present (how they affect others and are affected by them, for good or bad, today).

Some sociologists had also noted the bridging role of relationality, between the individual and society. Georg Simmel writing in the 1930s about city life noted that 'one nowhere feels as lonely and lost as in the metropolitan crowd'. Writing after the Second World War in the shadow of Nazism and Stalinism Hannah Arendt viewed loneliness as a societal trend and a sinister menace for humanity. Widespread loneliness and alienation in society could make people susceptible to the pull of totalitarianism. For her this was a political, not only a mental health, phenomenon and challenge. Here she comments:

> What prepares men (sic) for totalitarian domination in the non-totalitarian world is the fact that loneliness, once a borderline experience usually suffered in certain marginal social conditions like old age, has become an everyday experience of the ever-growing masses of our century.
>
> (Arendt 1951)

Before Arendt's version of pessimism about the human condition, Freud offered his own, which was that neurosis is the price we pay for living with the constraints imposed upon individuals in civilised societies (Freud 1930). Another psychoanalyst, Erich Fromm, argued that we can and should historicise Freud's generalisations and place them in particular social contexts (Fromm 1944). He and others in the early Frankfurt School explored the *particular* expectations imposed on citizens in this rather than that societal form. He contrasted the norms of consumer capitalism with those that might be achieved under a form of humanistic socialism. This theme of the vagaries of late capitalism, especially when it morphed into neoliberalism, became the interest of other social scientists who sought to provide the links that C.W. Mills was encouraging between private troubles and public issues (Wilkinson 2005).

The fear of being alone became linked to the failure of the emerging zeitgeist within American society of atomised individualism. Being alone was terrifying in the absence of a group or approved cause to acquiesce to and join, when people were under the cultural pressure of individualism to 'do their own thing in their own time'. If cancer was now the largest existential threat to citizens in bodily terms, then loneliness, was becoming a threat to the peace of mind of individuals (Reissman et al. 2001).

Thus the world of American capitalism was, from the Second World War on, a source of loneliness, but also a normative baseline measure of success for the individual citizen. Loneliness reflected social causes, such as atomisation in a competitive industrial society, but also a social judgment or 'emotion-rule' to comply with. The rise of consumerism, and its amplification after the 1980s, was the wider context in the West, led by the USA, for more prevalent forms of loneliness, to be both experienced and feared.

Other countries were to follow this American trend, albeit sometimes in less extreme form. The particular twist on anxiety suggested in its ubiquity by Freud, were new forms of competitiveness and a rejection and stigmatisation of those unable, or unwilling, to compete in a capitalist society. For example this applied to those unable or unwilling to work and so demonstrate personal autonomy. By contrast, those prepared to work hard might follow the American Dream and buy their way to happiness.

A US cohort study has demonstrated that the average US child growing up in the 1990s is much more likely than those from the 1950s, to be in a state of chronic anxiety (Twenge 2000). This is little surprising, as it is a reflection of a collective delusion under consumer capitalism, which is that the more people have, the happier they will be. Economists have now demonstrated this falsehood, created by the norms of consumerism and political scientists have noted how it turns adults into children (Barber 2008).

With these cultural points in mind, the earlier points about the ubiquity of our individual vulnerability to be distressed are also true and they may account for individual variability in resilience to cultural pressures. Anxiety is intrinsic to the human condition. However, in modern capitalist societies, with multiple concomitant threats to the self, relationships for some can invoke an overwhelming dread of others.

Social anxiety is, though, a continuum. Few of us are confident all of the time in all interpersonal contexts. Most of us find ways of coping with this fact. When in doubt, avoidance tends to be a first line of defence, if it is available. (The specific anxieties located at either end of the social ladder are discussed below.) People develop mental strategies, as well as routines to navigate their way with, or around, other people in public spaces. Reliable rhythms of movement and rest help people to cope with anxiety, though there are inequalities in this sort of control. Some, more than others, are obliged to enter public spaces. This variation is governed by considerations of both available time and money and is a fluxing and complex example of inequality. Those social anxieties are not only an individual impairment but they also reflect role differences and differences in social obligations.

Additionally when people move localities, change jobs, retire or get divorced, these points of transition may threaten personal security or provide liberating opportunities. This shifting and ambiguous relationship between inner security and outer changes can lead to some counter-intuitive outcomes. For example, although a common assumption is that 'winning the lottery' will change our lives for the better and substantially, there is no evidence that this is actually true in practice.

People employ socio-spatial practices and routines to manage anxieties. We like to know 'where we are' about daily life and the routines we prefer to manage it, in or out of our homes. The relationship between 'internal' mental habits and 'external' practice is reflected in everyday performances. One of these is moving around, such as walking and commuting, discussed in Chapter 5.

Routine habits of movement and rest tend to ingrain a sense of stability and security in the practice of everyday life. Disruptions of those habits increase the risk of anxiety emerging – hence why some people become homesick, even when on vacation. People seek to retain security, via their bodily routines. However, ageing and changing social contexts challenge their retention, creating anxiety and necessitating existential reflection. These fluctuations in self-confidence, and the inner reflections they might provoke, are not just intra-subjective phenomena, they always exist in relation to others, present or absent. Accordingly, our attention turns to social networks.

The recurring importance of social networks for managing anxiety and loneliness

As a psychosocial state, loneliness is transferable to others in social networks. Like other subjective states (such as happiness) it can be mediated through networks of interaction. The latter includes social contagion, as well as shared cultures and places. Social networks are created by social ties (with family, community members and significant others). They provide strategies for action and have the power to facilitate or restrict access to resources and forms of emotional or instrumental support.

Interpersonal ties provide a sense of belonging and shape our sense of identity. They are also sources of information and influence. Researchers of social capital focus on networks as resources in daily living. Social connectivity between people provides personal recognition and the advantages of acts of mutuality, which some social contexts encourage more than others. Putnam's classic study of social connectedness in modern American society points to the reduction in the regularity of friendship and neighbour contact (Putnam 2000).

Loneliness emerges from a reduction of conversational exchange in routine daily living and a loss of familiarity with and trust in, those around us. The lack of social cohesion and sense of belonging is accompanied by a sense of social alienation – a disconnection or distancing from previously held values, practices and relations with social groups in a community. Thus loneliness is not only the plight of an individual but a description of their social-psychological context and always implies the presence or absence of others. That general point is summarised here by Cacioppo et al.:

> Loneliness – is not only a function of the individual but is also a property of groups of people. People who are lonely tend to be linked to others who are lonely, an effect that is stronger for geographically proximal than distant friends yet extends up to three degrees of separation (friends' friends' friend) within the social network.
>
> (Cacioppo et al. 2009).

Social contagion (the spontaneous spread of behaviours and emotions through a network, with conscious and unconscious components) is one aspect of the spread of loneliness. Over time, loneliness establishes norms of negative social reactions, resulting in the loss of habitual social contact. Distancing from other people is provoked by the cognitive content of the social context of loneliness.

Shyness, anxiety, social awkwardness and 'homophily' (the choice to be with other like-minded lonely people) form the bases of a shared micro-social environment. Within the latter, connected individuals experience concomitant social exposure, which contributes to the spread of loneliness. This process may be reinforced by contexts of austerity and marginalisation. The link between private troubles and public issues is exemplified by lonely people in their social context. Their withdrawal and marginalisation, or rejection by others, then create a vicious cycle. It becomes a mechanism for the social reproduction of loneliness.

As well as social contagion, some researchers have focused on 'cognitive social capital', which refers to values, attitudes and beliefs accrued during our interactions with others (Coletta and Cullen 2002). As they emerge in relation to others, they imply the need to understand interpersonal trust and degrees of reciprocity. These can be extended to shared action, where people together participate in aspects of civil society (Harpham 2008); this is a collective activity described as 'structural social capital'. For example, participation in voluntary activity generates contingent forms of social integration for direct mutual benefit and that of their locality. Lonely people do not participate in this activity, though note in some contexts they may be its beneficiaries.

The level and degree of benefits to people of social contact involve a bridge between the inner lives and actions of individuals and their being with others. Others can provide us with information, enhance our autonomy, via affectional and supportive bonds, and they offer new opportunities, which cannot emerge from individual effort alone. This bridging function has invited a research emphasis on ties between us, which contingently might vary in their strength.

Both 'strong' and 'weak' ties are associated with lower levels of loneliness (Sandstrom and Wells 2014; Granovetter 1973). However, weak ties may have greater potential for addressing personal isolation, because they provide social opportunities, made possible by brief encounters with distal acquaintances (examples of this were given in Chapter 1). Whilst we usually are acculturated to believe that strong family loyalties are the optimal form of relationality, weak ties increase the likelihood of a respect for personal autonomy and are less stressful because of fewer expectations of reciprocal obligations (Rogers et al. 2014). Numerically, weak ties are multiple and fluid and have the advantage that they can peter out with few emotional consequences, which is not the case with blood ties.

Those who have access to, and resources for, social participation are likely to be less lonely than those without these situated opportunities. Those at the bottom of the socio-economic scale have fewer resources when responding to a state of loneliness. The self-confidence of lonely people increases the more that they participate in life and activities with others. Moreover, the contingent quantity and quality of community assets facilitate that participation. Localities, within which lonely people interact, are shaped and constrained by wider social and economic circumstances. For example, austerity undermines the availability of community assets, which in turn increases personally experienced stress or distress. Low levels of community resources in areas of deprivation mean that participation for lonely people is restricted from the 'supply side' and is not about individual effort or resilience (Ellis et al. 2020).

The technological shift to a digital age has promoted connectivity more than in the past and potentially provides the opportunity for participation online, as an alternative or addition to offline communities. Social media can at times be hostile and frightening, particularly exposing those, who are already psychologically vulnerable. They do put those already vulnerable to new risks of distress. However, when working well, digital relationships can be deployed to complement their absence in the offline world.

The downside is that online life can isolate people from face-to-face traditional relationships (Allen et al. 2020). However, they also enable the expression of feelings and set up beneficial conversations. For those who are alone or lonely online connectedness can provide cathartic release, as well as shape or model strategies for managing life. They can validate selfhood and create new ties, maybe building community sociability, through online disinhibition. The latter is the inverse of forms of social anxiety lonely people may manifest in situ with others. Online ties are flexible, can be kept at a distance, fleeting, characterised by an ease of negotiation and the convenience of opting out, when they are no longer working for the person (Nowland et al. 2018). To summarise here, our new digital age has brought with it both threats and opportunities to increase social connectivity and reduce loneliness.

Anxiety: tough at the top but worse at the bottom

Loneliness is predictive of anxiety (as well as depression). Loneliness increases feelings of perceived isolation, which leads to feelings of separation anxiety (Owczarek et al. 2022). The experience of anxiety is articulated differently according to social position and links with the gradient of inequality.

The case that the poorest are most at risk of loneliness and ordinary distress in society is clear. Higher rates of diagnosed anxiety disorders are indicative of, and causally linked to, the higher prevalence of social isolation and its health burden in lower socio-economic groups. Residents of deprived neighbourhoods are more likely to be lonely than those in better off ones (Algren et al. 2020).

However, unequal societies bring with them challenges to the self, whatever a person's position or neighbourhood. To recognise that one is at a point in a hierarchy, brings with it the challenge of maintaining that position and fear of losing it. It can also invoke aspirations for wealth and upward social mobility. Michael Marmot in his book *Status Syndrome* (Marmot 2004) illuminates the psychosocial effects of status comparisons linked to income inequality.

Low-inequality countries report less status anxiety than those in higher-inequality countries, which is linked to status competition, and the sense of inferiority of those with less social status. Economic inequality makes people feel that they live in a society where they are constantly concerned and competing with each other for their status and personal recognition. Thus, income inequality increases status anxiety for everyone, not just those who are poor, though the latter have the additional burden of consumerist pressures that are unaffordable.

In very poor countries there may be absolute poverty and basic needs for food, water, income and shelter jeopardise the physical and mental health of those affected (Sennett and Cobb 1972; Doyal and Gough 1991). In countries with a welfare safety net, those with poor task control, job security, pension rights or trade union protection will still encounter subjective insecurity, as a function of external unpredictability. For this reason, in developed countries, poorer-paid workers in insecure employment, making social comparisons with the better-off around them, tend to have poorer mental health. This trend was evident, even *prior* to the emergence of neoliberal reforms in the 1980s and the downturn of the capitalist economy in 2008 (Power et al. 2015).

After those changes, the tendency was amplified, as trade union protections weakened and new norms of the 'gig economy' emerged. These changes differentially impact on younger workers, whose average job security and access to the housing market have compared less favourably to their parents' generation (Ferrante et al. 2019). Thus, wherever we are in the hierarchy of status and wealth in unequal societies, at a point in time, as individuals we may have had adverse or propitious circumstances in our upbringing. Those vulnerabilities of childhood inflect our security (more on this in the next chapter).

What's love got to do with it?

We tend to thrive in loving relationships and we all have a need to receive and give love in its various forms. For example, we pine for lost loved ones and we suffer the emotional legacy of emotional neglect in our childhoods. The applied philosopher Alain De Botton makes the point that love is not just a subjective emotion. It also has symbolic value as a communication in relation to others. It has both a performative aspect and assumes an on-looking audience, actual or imagined. It matters to us what others think of us and so social value is bound up with love:

> with the amount of love we stand to receive as a consequence of high status Money, fame and influence may be valued more as tokens of – and as means to – love rather than as ends in themselves.
>
> (De Botton 2004)

This also raises recurring questions about inner feelings of respect and recognition, and the circumstances under which they emerge and are maintained, as well as the opposite side of the same coin which entails abuse, hate, betrayal and humiliation. Simply *having* a high status increases the chances of respect and recognition. The inverse is also true: having a low status increases the risk of social defeat and personal demoralisation. Those rich financially and psychologically will be more likely to experience the world as pleasant and meaningful. Those who are poor financially and psychologically are more likely to lack value in the eyes of others, and they are more likely to doubt themselves and act out in self-defeating or dysfunctional ways. That vulnerability to experienced and enacted distress is not just a personal tendency for some individuals more than others, it is also more likely to become evident in periods of social dislocation and threat.

Being financially well off but still being anxious

Robert Frank, in his book *Richistan* (2008), notes two richer groups, which are vulnerable to anxiety. The first is the simply 'well off' nouveau riche, who feel precarious about maintaining their newly acquired luxuries. This turns them typically (but not inevitably) into aggressive reactionaries, who celebrate their individual efforts and are disdainful of their feckless poorer peers. 'Bootstrap individualism' might characterise their thoughts and actions. However, they worry constantly about the material gains they have achieved from individual struggle, but which now might be lost.

The second is the very rich (the interpersonal field of which is explored darkly in TV series such as *Succession* and *White Lotus*). Frank discusses how their butlers are trained to anticipate an employer's every whim and cites a warning piece of wisdom to these trainees. This comes from the chief instructor of the 'butler boot camp':

> They're health freaks ... These people are very successful and guess what, they want to live forever. These are very germ-orientated people. Get used to it, germs are *huge* in this world.

The last sentence refers not to the world of humanity as a whole, but the particular world of the super-rich. The class gradient in both morbidity and mortality is clear: the poor are sicker and die younger. However, when it comes to ontological security or existential anxiety, little is gained by being beyond a certain level of income.

Basically, up to a point, people are happier the more money they have but the benefits of wealth then soon diminish. This has become known as the 'Easterlin Paradox': as we become richer we do not necessarily become happier, which is demonstrated recurrently in longitudinal data (Easterlin 1974). The Scandinavian countries, with their social democratic history, relative absence of involvement in war, good welfare systems and anti-materialistic norms have tended to be the happiest, since the Second World War. However, some much poorer nations in Central and South America, with significantly lower GDPs, may sometimes compare favourably. For example, poorer Catholic countries tend to 'punch above their weight' in the trend.

Part of the Easterlin Paradox is that those who are well off, in richer countries, such as the USA, do not seem to be any happier than those who are poorer than them. One factor, already mentioned, is anxiety of loss. Wealth can be lost as well as gained and, linked to this, there is the matter of status. If wealth brings a particular cultural expectation of standing in a community, then the performativity of that status has to be maintained. Should money be flaunted or hidden? How should those with money present themselves to their peers? This matter of 'keeping up appearances' is an ongoing source of anxiety for these social actors.

Another factor is the cognitive dissonance that might be around in some upwardly mobile rich people about the comforts of their earlier simpler life. For some, there are other personal stressors. Should they give their excess of money away and, if so, to whom and on what basis? Might their children who have known nothing but opulence behave in ways that are selfish, reckless or disappointing because of their lack of the need to try hard and responsibly in life? This fear of a 'spoilt brat' scenario can prompt some rich people to deny their children access to resources or make them attend boot camps, in order to put them in touch with ordinary stressors in life.

At the other end of the social scale in developed societies, which see little absolute poverty compared to the least developed, there are other challenges. These include the working poor who still cannot afford their regular household bills. (In the UK in recent times some dual-income families still have had to resort to food banks, despite living in a welfare economy.) These stressors can create anxiety, envy and shame for some individuals.

The shame that might be experienced by the working poor and the guilt that might be experienced by their observing neighbours is more likely with physical proximity. In large cities, the rich and poorer people tend to live cheek by jowl. They observe one another as neighbours and in common public places, as when the well-healed walk past homeless people. Poorer neighbours look on to richer ones with a mixture of envy and intrigue about a better life.

In smaller towns, demographic differentiations of housing might separate these groups more. However, in large cities, like London, the co-existence of wealth and want produces emotional reactions across the class divide. Even in the rich locales of Mayfair and Richmond, shops must be staffed and homes, offices and streets need to be cleaned. This enmeshment of the classes in particular places produces emotional impacts for everyone. Being rich brings its problems. Being poor brings even more. When they live nearby, then other problems of envy and guilt also emerge, when social comparisons are part of daily life, whether or not they are consciously acknowledged.

Conclusion

Loneliness and anxiety are part of the human condition and they are linked inextricably to health and well-being. Though part of our species' character, they are inflected by particular social conditions, within and across time and space. We have tried to depict that biopsychosocial intersection and its complexities above. Loneliness has had a long history of being framed variously in existential, medical and social-scientific terms. Different starting points contribute to diverse ways of understanding the genesis, outcomes, amelioration and socially patterned experiences of living with loneliness.

Anxiety, depression and loneliness both reflect and maintain inequalities. The experience of heightened rates of distress and loneliness, in different groups within society, belies the truism that social status is simply good for the rich. It is much more complex than this, as we showed above. We continue in the next two chapters to look at the uneven distribution of suffering and changes of risk across the lifespan.

References

Arendt, H. 1951. *The Origins of Totalitarianism*. London: Penguin Classics.

Alberti, F. 2019. *A Biography of Loneliness: The History of an Emotion*. Oxford: Oxford University Press.

Algren, M.H., O. Ekholm, L. Nielsen, A.K. Ersbøll, C. K. Bak, and P.T. Andersen. 2020. "Social Isolation, Loneliness, Socioeconomic Status, and Health-Risk Behaviour in Deprived Neighbourhoods in Denmark: A Cross-Sectional Study." *Social Science & Medicine: Population Health* 10: 100546.

Allen, C., I. Vassilev, A. Kennedy, and A. Rogers. 2020. "The Work and Relatedness of Ties Mediated Online in Supporting Long-Term Condition Self-Management." *Sociology of Health & Illness* 42 (3): 579–595.

Allport, G.W. 1968. *The Person in Psychology*. Boston, MA: Beacon Press.

Barbek, R.M.E., A.C. Makowski, and O. von dem Knesebeck. 2021. "Social Inequalities in Health Anxiety: A Systematic Review and Meta-analysis." *Journal of Psychosomatic Research* 153: 110706.

Barber, B.R. 2008. *"Consumed" How Markets Corrupt Children, Infantilize Adults and Swallow Citizens Whole*. New York: Norton.

Binnie, J., J. Holloway, S. Millington, and C. Young. 2007. "Mundane Geographies: Alienation, Potentialities and Practice." *Journal of Environment & Planning* 39 (3), 515–520.

Bosma, H., M. Jansen, S. Schefman, K.J. Hajema, and F. Feron. 2015. "Lonely at the Bottom: A Cross-Sectional Study on Being Ill, Poor, and Lonely." *Public Health* 129 (2): 185–187.

Bourdieu, P. 1984. *Distinction: A Social Critique of the Judgment of Taste*. London: Routledge.

Bowlby, J. 1951. *Maternal Care and Mental Health*. Geneva: World Health Organization.

Cacioppo, J.T., J.H. Fowler, and N.A. Christakis. 2009. "Alone in the Crowd: The Structure and Spread of Loneliness in a Large Social Network." *Journal of Personality & Social Psychology* 97 (6): 977–91.

Child, S.T., and L. Lawton. 2019. "Loneliness and Social Isolation among Young and Late Middle-age Adults. Associations with Personal Networks and Social Participation." *Aging & Mental Health* 23 (2): 196–204.

Colletta, N.J., and M.L. Cullen. 2002. "Social Capital and Social Cohesion: Case Studies from Cambodia and Rwanda." In *The Role of Social Capital in Development: An Empirical Assessment*, edited by C. Grootaert and T.van Bastelaer, 21–31. Cambridge: Cambridge University Press.

Das-Munshi, J., D. Goldberg, P.E. Bebbington, D.K. Bhugra, T.S. Brugha, M.E. Dewey, R. Jenkins, R. Stewart, and M. Prince. 2008. "Public Health Significance of Mixed Anxiety and Depression: Beyond Current Classification." *The British Journal of Psychiatry* 192 (3): 171–177.

De Botton, A. 2004. *Status Anxiety*. London: Hamilton.

Delanty, G. 2003. *Community*. London: Routledge.

Doyal, L., and I. Gough. 1991. *A Theory of Human Need*. Basingstoke: Palgrave.

Easterlin, R. 1974. "Does Economic Growth Improve the Human Lot? Some Empirical Evidence." In *Nations and Households in Economic Growth: Essays in Honor of Moses Abramovitz*, edited by P.A. David and M.W. Reder, 12–20. New York: Academic Press, Inc.

Eckhard, J. 2018. "Does Poverty Increase the Risk of Social Isolation? Insights Based on Panel Data from Germany." *The Sociological Quarterly* 59 (2): 338–359.

Ellis, J., R. Band, K. Kinsella, T. Cheetham-Blake, E. James, S. Ewings, and A. Rogers. 2020. "Optimising and Profiling Pre-implementation Contexts to Create and Implement a Public Health Network Intervention for Tackling Loneliness." *Implementation Science: IS* 15 (1): 35.

Ferrante, G., F. Fasanelli, A. Gigantesco, et al. 2019. "Is the Association between Precarious Employment and Mental Health Mediated by Economic Difficulties in Males? Results from Two Italian Studies." *BMC Public Health* 19 (1): 869.

Frank, R. 2008. *Richistan: A Journey through the American Wealth Boom and the Lives of the New Rich*. London: Penguin Random House.

Freud, S. 1930. *Civilisation and Its Discontents*, translated by J. Strachey. London: Hogarth Press.

Freud, S. 1917. "Trauer und Melancholie." *Internationale Zeitschrift für Ärztliche Psychoanalyse* 4: 288–301.

Fromm, E. 1944. "Individual and Social Origins of Neurosis." *American Sociological Review* 9 (4): 10–15.

Granovetter, M.S. 1973. "The Strength of Weak Ties." *American Journal of Sociology* 78 (6): 1360–1380.

Grøn, A. 2008. *The Concept of Anxiety in Søren Kierkegaard*, translated by J. B. L. Knox. Macon: Mercer University Press.

Kearns, A., E. Whitley, C. Tannahill, and A. Ellaway. 2015. "Loneliness, Social Relations and Health and Well-Being in Deprived Communities." *Psychology, Health & Medicine* 20 (3): 332–344.

Lasgaard, M., K. Friis, and M. Shevlin. 2016. "'Where are all the lonely people?' A Population-Based Study of High-Risk Groups across the Life Span." *Social Psychiatry & Psychiatric Epidemiology* 51 (10): 1373–1384.

Hansen, T., and B. Slagsvold. 2016. "Late-Life Loneliness in 11 European Countries: Results from the Generations and Gender Survey." *Social Indicators Research* 129 (1): 445–464.

Layard, R. 2005. *Happiness*. London: Penguin.

Marmot, M. 2004. *Status Syndrome: How Your Social Standing Directly Affects Your Health and Life Expectancy*. London: Bloomsbury.

Neilson, D. 2015. "Class, Precarity, and Anxiety under Neoliberal Global Capitalism: From Denial to Resistance." *Theory & Psychology* 25 (2): 184–201.

Pilgrim, D., A. Rogers, and R.P. Bentall. 1999. "The Medicalisation of Misery: A Critical Realist Analysis of the Concept of Depression." *Journal of Mental Health* 8 (3): 261–274.

Power, E., M. Clarke, I. Kelleher, H. Coughlan, F. Lynch, D. Connor, C. Fitzpatrick, M. Harley, and M. Cannon. 2015. "The Association between Economic Inactivity and Mental Health among Young People: A Longitudinal Study of Young Adults Who Are Not in Employment, Education or Training." *Irish Journal of Psychological Medicine* 32 (1): 155–160. doi: 10.1017/ipm.2014.85.

Hansen, N., and C. Philo. 2007. "The Normality of Doing Things Differently: Bodies, and Disability Geography." *Tijdschrift Voor Economische en Sociale Geografie* 98 (4): 493–506. doi: 10.1111/j.1467-9663.2007.00417.x.

Harpham, T. 2008. "The Measurement of Community Social Capital through Surveys." In *Social Capital and Health*, edited by I. KawachI, S.V. Subramanian and D. Kim, 70–82. New York: Springer.

Holt-Lunstad, J., T.B. Smith, M. Baker, T. Harris, and D. Stephenson. 2015. "Loneliness and Social Isolation as Risk Factors for Mortality: A Meta-analytic Review." *Perspectives on Psychological Science* 10 (2): 227–237.

Lochner, K., I. Kawachi, and B.P. Kennedy. 1999. "Social Capital: A Guide to Its Measurement." *Health & Place* 5 (4): 259–270.

Hochschild, A. 1983. *The Managed Heart: The Commercialization of Human Feeling*. Berkeley: University of California Press.

McHugh Power, J., C. Hannigan, P. Hyland, S. Brennan, F. Kee, and B.A. Lawlor. 2020. "Depressive Symptoms Predict Increased Social and Emotional Loneliness in Older Adults." *Aging & Mental Health* 24 (1): 110–118.

McKenna-Plumley, P.E., J.M. Groarke, R.N. Turner, and K. Yang. 2020. "Experiences of Loneliness: A Study Protocol for a Systematic Review and Thematic Synthesis of Qualitative Literature." *Systematic Reviews* 9 (1): 284.

Mills, C.W. 1959. *The Sociological Imagination*. Oxford: Oxford University Press.

Norton, P.J., and D.J. Paulus. 2017. "Transdiagnostic Models of Anxiety Disorder: Theoretical and Empirical Underpinnings." *Clinical Psychology Review* 56, 122–137.

Nowland, R., E.A. Necka, and J.T. Cacioppo. 2018. "Loneliness and Social Internet Use: Pathways to Reconnection in a Digital World?." *Perspectives on Psychological Science* 13 (1): 70–87.

Owczarek, M., E. Nolan, M. Shevlin, S. Butter, T. Karatzias, O. McBride, J. Murphy, F. Vallieres, R. Bentall, A. Martinez, and P. Hyland. 2022. "How Is Loneliness Related to Anxiety and Depression: A Population-Based Network Analysis in the Early Lockdown Period." *International Journal of Psychology* 57 (5): 585–596.

Peplau, L.A., and D. Perlman. 1982. "Perspectives on Loneliness." In *Loneliness: A Sourcebook of Current Theory, Research and Therapy*, edited by L.A. Peplau and D. Perlman, 1–18. New York: Wiley.

Pescosolido, B.A. 2006. "Of Pride and Prejudice: The Role of Sociology and Social Networks in Integrating the Health Sciences." *Journal of Health & Social Behavior* 47 (3): 189–208.

Putnam, R.D. 2000. *Bowling Alone: The Collapse And Revival Of American Community*. New York: Simon & Schuster.

Riesman, D., N. Glazer, and R. Denney. 2001. *The Lonely Crowd: A Study of the Changing American Character*. Yale: Yale University Press.

Rogers, A., I. Vassilev, A. Kennedy, C. Blickem, D. Reeves, and H. Brooks. 2014. "Why Less May Be More?: A Mixed Methods Study of the Work and Relatedness of 'Weak' Ties in Supporting Long Term Condition Self- Management." *Implementation Science* 9.

Rosen, G. 1968. *Madness in Society*. New York: Harper.

Sandstrom, G.M., and E.W. Dunn. 2014. "Social Interactions and Well-Being: The Surprising Power of Weak Ties." *Personality & Social Psychology Bulletin* 40 (7): 910–922.

Salway, S., E. Such, L. Preston, A. Booth, M. Zubair, C. Victor, and R. Raghavan. 2020. "Reducing Loneliness among Migrant and Ethnic Minority People: A Participatory Evidence Synthesis." 8 (10): 10.

Schirmer, W., and D. Michailakis. 2016. "Loneliness Among Older People as a Social Problem: The Perspectives of Medicine, Religion and Economy." *Ageing & Society* 36 (8): 1559–1579.

Sennett, R., and J. Cobb. 1972. *The Hidden Injuries of Class*. Cambridge: Cambridge University Press.

Scheid, T.L., and C. Anderson. 1995. "Living with Chronic Mental Illness: Understanding the Role of Work." *Community Mental Health Journal* 31 (2): 163–176.

Slee, A., I. Nazareth, N. Freemantle, and L. Horsfall. 2021. "Trends in Generalised Anxiety Disorders and Symptoms in Primary Care: UK Population-Based Cohort Study." *The British Journal of Psychiatry* 218 (3): 158–164.

Twenge, J.M. 2000. "The Age of Anxiety? Birth Cohort Change in Anxiety and Neuroticism, 1952–1993." *Journal of Personality & Social Psychology* 79 (6): 1007–1021. doi: 10.1037//0022-3514.79.6.1007. PMID: 11138751.

Tyrer, P. 2022. *Neurosis: Understanding Common Mental Illness*. Cambridge: Cambridge University Press.

van Tilburg, T.G. 1990. "The Size of the Supportive Network in Association with the Degree of Loneliness." In *Social Network Research: Substantive Issues and Methodological Questions*, edited by C.P.M. Knipscheer and T.C. Antonucci, 137–150. Lisse, The Netherlands: Swets & Zeitlinger.

Vassilev, I., A. Rogers, C. Sanders, S. Cheraghi-Sohi, C. Blickem, H. Brooks, D. Kapadia, D. Reeves, T. Doran, and A. Kennedy. 2014. "Social Status and Living with a Chronic Illness: An Exploration of Assessment and Meaning Attributed to Work and Employment." *Chronic Illness* 10 (4): 273–290.

Victor, C.R., and K. Yang. 2012. "The Prevalence of Loneliness among Adults: A Case Study of the United Kingdom." *The Journal of Psychology* 146 (1–2): 85–104.

Weiss, R.S. 1973. *Loneliness: The Experience of Emotional and Social Isolation*. Cambridge, MA: The MIT Press.

Wellman, B. 2001. The Persistence and Transformation of Community: From Neighbourhood Groups to Social Networks. Report to the Law Commission of Canada. Wellman Associates.

Winnicott, D.W. 1958. "The Capacity to Be Alone." In *The Maturational Processes and the Facilitating Environment*. London: Hogarth/Institute of Psycho-Analysis. Reprinted from *International Journal of Psycho-Analysis* 39 (5): 416–420.

Winnicott, D.W. 1957. *The Child and the Family*. London: Tavistock.

Wilkinson, R.G. 2005. *The Impact of Inequality: How to Make Sick Societies Healthier*. London: Routledge.

Wright, K. 2016. "Social Networks, Interpersonal Support and Health Outcomes: A Healthcommunication Perspective." *Frontiers in Communication* 1: 10.

7 Normal and abnormal suffering

Introduction

As the graffiti tells us: 'You are born, it's horrible and then you die'. The uneven distribution of experienced suffering, while we are alive, is the concern of this chapter. Life is more or less 'horrible' for people. Without that consideration of inequality, blanket offers of remediation, such as the panaceas of 'mindfulness' and 'acceptance', can obscure injustice.

This chapter considers three main questions. First, how is everyday suffering shaped by a class-divided society? Second, what inequalities in suffering are shaped by those experiencing trauma and those who do not? Third, how do those labelled as being psychologically abnormal, experience and adapt to their social rejection and the constraints on their citizenship? Answering these experiential questions extends the insight from Buddhism that suffering is 'built in' to being alive for everyone. We may all suffer but some of us are luckier than others in our lives about its salience, type and frequency. For example, generally it is easier to rejoice in the tent of plenty.

The theme of being in the same boat of human suffering, and yet some of us having a seat with a more comforting view, was obvious in relation to the recent Covid-19 pandemic. Under 'lockdown', city living in a small flat with small children was tougher to cope with than for those with large houses and spacious gardens. Extending this metaphor, maybe people are actually in different boats and suffering *is the sea*, which in different times and places is more or less rough, as they sail from birth to death. What is clear is that if suffering is certainly a shared human condition, then it is neither standardised in degree, nor is it distributed in equal measure.

An alternative starting point to discuss this co-presence of the ubiquity of suffering and its uneven distribution is developmental psychology. The newborn is thrown into the world with unequal chances. From conception onwards these are set by uterine conditions, we are not merely born unequal we are *conceived* that way, as second-wave feminist critiques of patriarchy note. And environmental impacts begin in utero, as the development of intelligence and the afflictions of congenital opiate or alcohol addiction demonstrate (May et al. 2018; Ross et al. 2015). At birth, our sex, ethnicity and the class of our parents, already cue what and how we might suffer in

DOI: 10.4324/9781003025641-7

our life to come. Subsequently, the quality of care in the early years varies and so has an uneven impact. Also, whether our embedding society is at war or peace will have substantially different implications for the young. The psychosocial context of human suffering is relevant then from conception to death.

For one version of developmental psychology, psychoanalysis, both its basic insights and the disputes amongst its enthusiasts are helpful to consider. The battle to preserve the ego, free from anxiety, begins in infancy. By the time we are adults, we have learned to defend ourselves in our particular ways, against both inner and outer threats to our secure sense of self. That natural human defensiveness, according to psychoanalysts, makes us all ill in our own particular way. The term 'personal psychopathology' is used in this tradition to indicate this point, no exceptions. For most of us this is what Erich Fromm (1955) called the 'pathology of normalcy'. When our defences succeed, then the insights of Buddhism about suffering are reminders of our impermanence and uneven life chances. When they fail then we become personally distressed and socially dysfunctional.

For Freud, anxiety was the price paid for living in a rule-bound society (Freud 1930). Societies are not all the same but they do expect conformity to rules as we are an interdependent species, a point noted in the previous chapter and to be picked up more below. For some writers, under the combined sway of Freud and Marx, the Frankfurt School, it was the complex relationship between psychopathology and contingent social conditions that was important to understand. The School was founded in 1923 and led after 1931 by Max Horkheimer, who posed the following long complex question, of relevance still today:

> What connections can be established in a specific social group, in a specific period in time, in specific countries, between the group the changes in the psychic structure of its individual members and the thoughts and institutions that are a product of that society, and that have, as a whole a formative effect upon the group under consideration?
>
> (Horkheimer 1931, 14)

Answering that complex question is not easy and requires recurring cautions about what is happening in particular contexts. What is clear though is that those contexts are always characterised by human relationships.

The centrality of relationships in accounting for differences in mental health status

Our sociability and interdependency as a mammalian species offer all societies the prospect of mutual care in principle. Both common empathy and the seeds of daily deliberative democracy come with that interdependency. Those seemingly positive and comforting aspects of our species are offset though by three personal disadvantages, which encourage suffering or make it difficult to deal with a society.

First, what if some individuals are very frightened of their fellows? What then? Does profound shyness become an illness? Are those preferring their own company rather than that of others betraying an obligation bequeathed to our species by evolution? Should they be pitied or condemned?

Second, once humans moved from being hunter-gatherers to becoming settled farmers and hunters, with territorial boundaries to defend, a weapon-using warring species was created (as remains evident today). That had consequences for our mental health at the level of individuals experiencing armed tribal, civil or international conflicts. To complement this inequality-inducing point about war, those evading the impact of armed conflicts have been *advantaged* psychologically. The trauma of war sets up the scenario of a particular form of inequality, with several consequences to be considered below for those affected, including even subsequent generations.

Third, interpersonal dependency, from cradle to grave, also brings with it a social *obligation* or perennial meta-rule in all human societies: by the time we reach maturity we must be socially accountable for our actions. If that basic social contract is broken then this can lead to the emergence of psychological states that are deemed to be abnormal and, with that, a particular form of inequality emerges. Moreover, as will be clear when discussing child sexual abuse below, interdependency also means that intimate contact with others may be detrimental to our mental health (Sartre's notion that 'hell is other people').

Social causes and social norms

If suffering is influenced by a range of biological, psychological and social factors (a point about causation) then its meaning is judged by professionals and laypeople alike in a normative context (a point about value judgments). For example, in today's psychiatric parlance, people who are frightened of others are suffering from 'social anxiety' and if that is chronic, this becomes re-framed as 'avoidant personality disorder' (Lane 2008). However, the monk in a silent order in his prayer cell has a socially sanctioned and even venerated way of living. One person's psychiatric diagnosis might be another's job description.

This reminds us that diagnostic labelling always reflects norms (Scheff 1966). However, to our knowledge, no society has been indifferent to those who are unusually fearful, sad, unintelligible or incorrigible. What societies have varied in historically, is the social relevance of this list and the explanations offered to account for it. Today we call it all 'mental disorder' but this is relatively recent. For example, by the 1960s, some psychiatrists distinguished and separated 'the neuroses' from 'true mental illnesses' and from 'abnormal developments of the personality' (Fish 1968).

The porous boundary between normality and abnormality is evident to us in everyday life. For example, when does sadness become clinical depression

(Horwitz and Wakefield 2007)? The diagnosis of any form of personality disorder has been particularly contentious. However, the very diverse range of symptoms described are basically chronic versions of distress, oddity or immorality. All of these long-term and self-preoccupied personality features merge into normal conduct at times. Returning to a point just made, about diagnoses and job descriptions, the diligent and successful accountant may be constantly sweating with symptoms of obsessive-compulsive disorder (Berrios 1988) and the self-confident CEO may have a very high psychopathy rating, just like the swaggering career criminal (Babiak and Hare 2007).

These examples suggest that judgements about abnormality always occur in a particular context. Given this point, the detrimental social impact of psychological abnormality remains open to debate. For example, extreme abnormality is linked to troublesome conduct – mad people are frightening and those diagnosed with a 'personality disordered' are incorrigible and so might be experienced by those in intimate contact as being burdensome and 'high maintenance'. But compare these troubling daily encounters to the havoc wreaked by the industrial–military complex, run by people who are allegedly completely sane and normal. The risks and disruption created to human welfare by those deemed to be mentally abnormal, by peers and professionals alike, shade into insignificance in this comparison to the impact of the destructive actions of those considered to be perfectly sane.

This ambiguity about psychological normality and abnormality reminds us of the need to consider both causes and meanings (which include our value judgments), while recognising that, at times, the latter might also have causal powers. Value judgments have causal powers in response to those who are labelled as being psychologically abnormal. Those judgments can determine who is granted citizenship and who is not, especially when legal powers are generated to ensure this division. Thus, both causes and meanings are woven through our relationships with others. For this reason, relationality is an important consideration, when offering holistic accounts of suffering and its varied distribution in human societies (Pilgrim et al. 2009).

To be clear, relationality is not *all important* because disparities of economic power and the biological constraints of our bodies and our unique powers of agency of decision-making also shape suffering. Put differently relationality is a necessary, but not a sufficient, basis for explanation; a point also true for the other planes of reality listed. Reality is laminated and these four planes (the natural world, relationality, social structures and our unique personalities) need to be considered in their totality and in interaction (Bhaskar 2008). This consideration of complexity in open human systems is explored further now, starting with the psychosocial implications of living in a class-divided society.

The hidden injuries of class

Poverty is a good overall predictor of poor physical and mental health. However, much more is needed to be said on psychosocial mediating processes, in order to account for the fact that some poor people live long, healthy and happy lives and some rich people do not.

Richard Sennett is a political scientist who has examined the fine-grain implications of living in a divided society (Sennett and Cobb 1972; Sennett 2003). At the centre of Sennett's work is a sensibility about the psychosocial aspects of social structures. How does class inequality impact the psyche of ordinary citizens? The response from Sennett and Cobb guides us in answering this question:

> Class society takes away from all the people within it the feeling of secure dignity in the eyes of others and of themselves. It does so in two ways: first, by the images it projects of why people belong to high or low classes – class presented as the ultimate outcome of personal ability; second, by the definition the society makes of the actions to be taken by people of any class to validate their dignity – legitimizations of self which do not, cannot work and so reinforce the original anxiety. The result of this, we believe, is that the activities which keep people moving in a class society, which make them seek more money, more possessions, higher-status jobs, do not originate in a materialistic desire, or even sensuous appreciation, of things, but out of an attempt to restore a psychological deprivation that the class structure has effected in their lives. In other words, *the psychological motivation instilled by a class society is to heal a doubt about the self rather than create more power over things and other persons in the outer world.*
>
> (Sennett and Cobb 1972, 170–171)

In his work on the corrosion of character in work and on welfare (the later book *Respect: The Formation of Character in an Age of Inequality*) Sennett returns to themes of both alienation and resilience for those who lack wealth, talent or both.

Employees may try and fail to restore a sense of equal participation and community in the workplace but are often left frustrated. The favoured notion of 'team work' succeeds for some people some of the time but not all people all of the time. The various personal tactics we might pursue to resist this continuation of Marx's original notion of alienation may be creative (Sennett himself favours music making) or dysfunctional (e.g., criminal and non-criminal expressions of greed and dominance over others).

Here Sennett notes that the worker in modern capitalism has to respond in some way or other to:

> the uncertainties of flexibility; the absence of deeply rooted trust and commitment; the superficiality of teamwork; most of all, the spectre of failing to make something of oneself in the world, to 'get a life' through one's work. All these conditions impel people to look for some other scene of attachment and depth.
>
> (Sennett 1998, 138)

The mental health implications of this ambiguous interaction between human agency, under conditions of unique biographical constraint, and the slow moving or immutable shared context of inequality are highly varied. That variation in open human systems, including those shaped by the vagaries under capitalism of class divisions, goes some way to account for why the linear tendency of the most poor in society being unhappy, unhealthy and dying younger is just that (a tendency, not a world of tramline social determinism). Other prospects under late capitalism to resist its emotional constraints and its threat, to meaning and our ontological security, have been explored by other social scientists, especially in the Frankfurt School tradition noted above (Habermas 1989; Fromm 1944).

For example, the British sociologists Stanley Cohen and Laurie Taylor famously documented 'escape attempts' (Cohen and Taylor 1992), which are the various ways we preserve our sanity and express our enjoyment and creativity, despite the external constraints of making a living and surviving daily life. This signals that human agency and constraining social (and biological structures) co-exist and are played out in a range of ways in open human systems, which are unequal in character. People cannot ultimately defy those constraints: in the end we are all dead and some of the time circumstances defy our agency or will. However, individuals can make the best of the hand of cards dealt to them from birth onwards.

Moreover, the particular character of those constraints of inequality varies over time and space. The limitations on mental health in a war zone are tighter and more oppressive than in peacetime. The longing for community, out of the grasp of the individual inhabiting a socio-economic system that ultimately is indifferent to their fate, but remains pointedly interested in their powers of consumption, began to find a new expression in the 1980s. This is when the individualism encouraged by neoliberalism (both psychologically and commercially epitomised in the advertising slogan 'Because you're worth it') culminated in the safe platitudes of identity politics. With that came a targeted interest in the grey pound, the pink pound and the black dollar. Identities can be commodified and commercialised readily.

Group belonging could be ensured online in virtual communities, which has a clear upside for people's sense of self-confidence. However, there is a downside as out-group members can be disparaged. Social media are a precarious source of ontological security and the tendency is for mental health decrements not improvement for their participants. A problem (amongst many) with identity politics played out on new social media is that they set people against one another. This may give meaning to individuals but it undermines social solidarity with others, especially those who disagree with you and are not a member of your allotted or acquired social group.

What Sennett's work has opened up and has been explored by others preceding him and since is the fraught question of how on a daily basis we seek and gain personal recognition and respect when the system we live in is incorrigibly unequal. A later Frankfurt School writer, Axel Honneth, argues that social systems and their particular structural inequalities afford personal recognition unevenly. For Honneth (2007), respect is primarily an *emotion* (which precedes cognition). With that the important secondary emotions of compassion and sympathy flow. We intuitively feel safe with some people and not others, even (wisely or not) on first meeting, when we know little or nothing about them.

Finally, in relation to 'normal alienation' or Fromm's 'pathology of normalcy', we can distinguish broad claims for parity of participation, encouraged by the rhetorical ethos of representative democracies, with its lack of assurance in practice. As Nancy Fraser has pointed out, the principle of parity of participation is a starting point for experienced equality but that can only be ensured by wider social conditions of possibility. Identity politics have focused over-personally and moralistically on the aspiration but have backgrounded the supra-personal socio-economic requirements for its guarantee (Fraser 1997).

These reflections from a range of writers, about what Sennett and Cobb call the 'hidden injuries of class', are a good starting point to understand the topic of this chapter. Next, two other major differentiations in society about experienced suffering are considered, in relation to those suffering trauma and those socially excluded because of their mental state.

Some are more equal than others: the uneven incidence of trauma

The social psychiatrist Adolf Meyer, started a discussion about biopsychosocial accounts of human functioning (Engel 1980). Meyer introduced psychological and social layers of determination about our mental lives. By contrast, psychologists were late in the game to this discussion, in part because their discipline was a 'new kid on the block' and in part because they used limited and misleading closed system reasoning, such as experiments producing evidence not relevant to everyday life (Johnstone and Boyle 2018). What these more psychosocial approaches to mental abnormality have emphasised (contra older eugenic biological explanations or those from experimental psychology) is that what happens to people and the meanings they attribute to their experiences, especially in relation to adversity in childhood and even trauma in adulthood, are centrally important in explaining subjective distress and social dysfunction.

When we come to consider the way in which traumatic processes and events impact on us, the legacy of assumptions of psychological medicine is what we mainly have to work with. Since the nineteenth century, we have witnessed two main attempts to account for human distress ('neurosis'), unintelligible conduct ('psychosis') and incorrigibility ('personality disorder'). The first, within eugenic Western psychiatry, depicts all these forms of 'mental disorder' as wholly or largely genetically determined.

The second attempt has invoked a range of environmental explanations, some of which are seemingly at odds; the most obvious example in the twentieth century was the discrepant accounts from behaviourists and psychoanalysts. These frameworks of primary causation about normal and abnormal mental life (bio-determinism versus versions of environmentalism) are not without their competing merits, if judged by empirical evidence, but they might all claim a dubious preeminent explanatory role.

An obvious point then is that, in truth, we do not know *for certain* why this person in this context is manifesting conduct, which by the norms of their culture, might be called either normal or abnormal. There is a difference between a broad *rationale of explanation* and whether or not any such overarching guide provides us with *definitive answers* about why this person is acting and experiencing life in this rather than that way.

That question of 'this particular-person-in-this-particular-context' reasoning (pace Meyer) is relevant for both normal and abnormal psychology. For example, why are some poor people happy despite poverty creating a tendency for experiencing misery? Why do some people with a secure family life and adequate financial stability still experience distress or drink too heavily or commit suicide out of the blue? In other words, in open systems the best we can do is seek an understanding of particular lives and even that will be fraught with uncertainties. Good novelists and wise psychotherapists get to grips with that complexity and uncertainty and record its situated nuances. The biopsychosocial model is another pathway into grappling with these matters, though it is a model not a pan-explanatory theory, explaining everybody's personal functioning in all their circumstances (Pilgrim 2015).

Adversity, the biopsychosocial model and mind–body interactions

Trauma is an extreme event: an explosion for the combatant, the shock of those injured in a rail crash, the trapped victim of a fire or the child sexually violated etc. When trauma is placed in a wider context of adversity, then the biopsychosocial model invites us to challenge mind–body dualism and the simplistic division of mental and physical illness.

The latter division is often made in mainstream medicine and even by its internal critics. For example, Thomas Szasz, a psychiatrist, only considered physical conditions with biological signs as being real (Szasz 1961). By contrast, mental illnesses, he argued, were a myth and mystification, better framed as moral dilemmas or recurring 'problems of living'. They reflected micro-political power struggles, with symptom-formation reflecting defeat (learned helplessness) or at times an unconscious tactic to influence others. (Szasz was a psychoanalyst, so he was replaying here Freud's insight about the secondary gain of mental illness.)

The absence of biomarkers or biological aetiology was central to Szasz' argument. However, there are many physical conditions in which we do not understand their origins for certain. Take Type 1 diabetes; we understand how it develops in the body as certain cells in the pancreas stop working. Technically this is called the 'pathogenesis' of the condition. However, researchers still do not understand, for certain, its primary cause (or causes) – technically called 'aetiology'. This lack of clarity is then extended to what are called 'medically unexplained symptoms'. These raise more questions than answers. Is the patient faking or exaggerating their malaise for some sort of personal gain? Alternatively, what if their diagnosticians are simply missing a needed insight and the patient is being wrongly accused?

Also there are many examples of biopsychosocial interactions in relation to the co-dependence of physical health and psychological functioning. The chronic pain of arthritis is depressing and alters available social activity and contact. In the other direction, depressed people may harm their own physical health by neglectful personal habits and by resorting to the excessive use of alcohol. Both diabetes and cardiac disease often prompt low mood in patients and, in the other direction, depressive loss reactions increase the risk of heart attacks (Steptoe et al. 2007; Fowler and Christakis 2008).

Trauma in war and peace

The psychological and social aspects of adversity, and its acute version of trauma, are important aspects of the unequal experience of suffering in society. Much of the literature on this point is derived from psychiatric understandings of the psychological trauma experienced by combatants, beginning with descriptions during the First World War (Shephard 2002). 'Shellshock' gave way conceptually to 'war neurosis', 'battle stress' and now 'Post-traumatic Stress Disorder', which is normalised now in the vernacular as 'PTSD'.

The cultural challenge of accepting psychological trauma in society was revealed during the 1920s, when those affected but physically unharmed attempted to live ordinary lives. This picture of a hidden complex world of the survivors of war trauma recurred. By the second half of the twentieth century, civilians, not combatants, were numerically predominant victims. Those surviving the Nazi Holocaust, either at the opening of the death camps or displaced as refugees in anxious flight, were an early indicator of this more recent trend. Since then, the systematic bombing of unarmed civilians in, for example, Iraq, Syria and Ukraine confirms this point, that war trauma is no longer the narrow concern of military psychiatry.

It is not surprising then that a focus in the work of the child psychiatrist and psychoanalyst, John Bowlby, came to the fore at the end of the Second World War. His interest was in children's mental health and the role of disrupted attachments in their lives. It was displaced and traumatised children, not soldiers, now who invited a professional interest in trauma (Bowlby 1951). Apart from Bowlby's attachment theory beginning a new chapter in psychosocial reflections, in the wake of those from Freud and Meyer, it also was the basis for illuminating a new and often hidden occurrence of trauma. This was the contested matter of child sexual abuse and its traumatic consequences, which is considered more below.

War is not good for the mental health of people. Peaceful stability brings with it an existential anchor point in our lives, which is to be without the immediate fear of death and injury or the loss and injury of others. However, not all people living through wars suffer what in psychiatric terms is called, for now, PTSD. Some seem to be psychologically well-adjusted and others are affected more subtly in their lives and so they are 'below the radar' of professional surveillance and labelling.

For example, those previously temperamentally sociable may turn quietly away and say little when war is over but show no clear-cut psychological dysfunction. Others may become more gregarious or assertive to the point of aggressiveness, when dealing with others in their daily lives. Previously easy-going people may have become more suspicious of others, without manifesting full-blown paranoia. In other words trauma creates inequalities in a range of ways experientially, in those who may never present to professionals during the rest of their lives. The caution returns again at this point that suffering is best seen as a psychosocial continuum, not a definitive medical category.

A further psychosocial consequence of war trauma is in relation to the children of its survivors. Expectations of normality ascribed to them during a post-war period, alongside the narratives (or silences) of their parents affect their mental lives, consciously and unconsciously. They may internalise, in various ways, feelings of guilt, anger and loss from the generation above them. They may become more preoccupied earnestly by psychological and historical matters, compared to their peers with non-traumatised parents. War then shapes the psyche of more than its direct victims. Literature on the impact of trauma from one generation to another is summarised in Box 7.1.

Box 7.1 Transgenerational trauma

Trauma can leave a legacy for subsequent generations, seemingly themselves living now in benign circumstances. For example, this effect has been demonstrated in studies of the children of those surviving the Nazi Holocaust. The latter display a range of psychological characteristics from heightened resilience to life stressors, right through to transmitted post-traumatic symptoms. Lower self-rated health, poorer socio-economic status and higher rates of reported stress have been found among Palestinians displaced during the Nakba of 1948 and their descendants, in comparison to families who were not displaced. Elevated post-traumatic stress symptoms have been found among descendants of the Armenian genocide. Studies of Canadian First Nations indigenous peoples found that a family history of forced boarding school attendance and removal from one's family and community is associated with a number of subsequent behavioural challenges in later generations.

These include increased exposure to sexual violence, opiate use and a greater involvement in child welfare systems.

Past adversity combines with effects of daily indignities to affect the subjective sense of confidence and worth of marginalised groups of people, which might be coloured subjectively in some individuals by historical loss. Studies of First Nation North Americans indicate that this combination of factors manifests itself as an increased tendency to anxiety and substance misuse. Past and present subjectively interact recurrently. Their own cultural symbols sit alongside decaying surroundings as a reminder of oppression and loss created by White colonial intrusion.

Martin Luther King reminded civil rights protesters in the 1960s, that racism in the USA preceded slavery and reflected the genocidal decimation of indigenous people. That legacy today has culminated in a raised incidence of PTSD and other psychiatric diagnoses, as well as disruptions to family and parent–child relationships.

Habitus as a resource

A problem with a diagnostic starting point, when discussing traumatised generations, is that it might suggest that social processes affecting our emotional life apply only to mental ill-health emerging from recent trauma. However, psychological health is best seen within the more general processes of habitus.

The latter refers to the internalisation of dispositions and practices particular to our contingent culture. These are then manifest in culturally specific tastes and lifestyles. The latter term is typically used to differentiate *individuals*. However, habitus implies that these are shared features or tendencies in those acculturated in a particular time and place, with particular familial legacies. This means that current conditions of adversity or its opposite can be considered in relation to events distant in time and experienced by ancestors. For this reason, a focus on trauma within the lifespan is only one consideration. Direct appeals to the 'lived experience' of social actors, consciously remembered, may simply miss this complexity.

Our mental states are, in part, determined by events before our birth. And when they are inherited as part of habitus they may be replicated via parenting styles and family-specific narratives repeated from generation to generation. We can think of this as embodied social knowledge. This then sets up the conditions of intergenerational transmission, which is largely unconscious to particular social actors. However, there are patterns that connect through time that can be described by historians, anthropologists and family therapists as part of an 'ecology of mind' (Bateson 1980). These patterns are the basis of 'transgenerational haunting'.

For example, displaced families show evidence of the transgenerational impact of exposure to historical traumatic events, through continuing to live in oppressive social conditions that routinely trigger these cultural memories and habits, some of which are dysfunctional and linked to distress. In particular, a lifestyle dominated by a 'survival mode' becomes evident (Bezo and Maggi 2015). This includes risky health practices, shame, anxiety, the hoarding of, and overconsumption of food, adoption of authoritarian parenting styles, high emotional neediness and a low sense of community trust.

Having considered the direct and indirect effects of war trauma, we now return to the sexual victimisation of children in peacetime and the lessons it offers about experienced inequality.

Child sexual abuse

The evidence now is that psychiatric patients are disproportionately the survivors of what is technically described in the research literature as 'adverse childhood experiences'. This empirical evidence, still accumulating, reflected an elephant in the room for twentieth-century advocates of environmental determinism, from Ivan Pavlov and Sigmund Freud to Adolf Meyer and Burrhus Skinner.

Of these, Freud remains the most controversial. He began by simply recording the high incidence of incest reports in his client work. Taken aback and perplexed by the number of victims he was encountering (seemingly often at the hands of respectable fathers like himself) he changed his mind. Maybe children were not really being sexually victimised but instead their own sexual fantasies were at play.

Some psychoanalysts such as Sandor Ferenczi retained a traumatic explanation for neurosis, extending the role of incest to the experience of birth. His insistence about the role of early trauma was a major factor in his personal loss of friendship with Freud. This split extended to other prior loyalists such as Otto Rank, who allied with Ferenczi in claiming that the traumatic role of the birth experience underpinned many cases of mental abnormality in adulthood.

However, a new version of environmentalist explanation was to push back against what was seen as a betrayal of victims by Freud (Masson 1985). This was the increasing evidence that the sexual victimisation is real and impactful, occurring in families and in other settings (such as sports coaching, residential social work, scouting, schools, nurseries and religious institutions). The empirical picture of sexual abuse suggests that Freud's revised model and the claims of moral panic advocates were seriously faulty and that they have misled public assumptions and policy about the rarity of CSA. More recently the social epidemiology of CSA has become clearer.

This is what we know (summarised from Pilgrim (2018a)). CSA occurs in all social classes (unlike physical abuse which occurs more in poorer family settings). Most cases of CSA emerge in families, even though the image of ‘stranger danger’ is culturally common. Even outside of families, usually the victim is already known to the perpetrator (e.g., in schooling and youth work); sudden stranger rape is rare. About one-third of CSA occurs at the hands of other children, with the perpetrators themselves often acting out their own victimhood.

Though class does not predict CSA, sex does. Around 95% of perpetrators are male. The female minority of perpetrators contains a mixture of sole offenders and confederates of male abusers. Most victims in families are female but there is a slight male preponderance in extra-familial abuse. Perpetrators may accumulate hundreds of victims during their adult lives. The costs to the state (police, social work and healthcare time and resources) are part of the picture of estimating harm; society as a whole suffers from the impact of CSA not just its targeted child victims.

Estimates of the rate of CSA suggest around a nine-fold under-recording in the UK Children Commissioners Report (2016). The reasons for this include: fear of reporting by victims or its normalisation in their family; the difficulty in police investigations and prosecutions, because simple denials from the accused obscure events, which are private and historical; and the cultural tendency to presume that parents in the privacy of their own homes are caring of their young. The latter assumption about benign adult care is applied as well to those in adult roles of authority (teachers, sports coaches and residential social workers) or public esteem (priests, celebrities and pop stars).

Moral panic theory in sociology has obscured, not clarified, the rate of CSA in society. The evidence undermines the notion that there is a moral panic about CSA today. Indeed it is relevant to note that one of the seminal figures in moral panic theory, Stanley Cohen, by the end of his life was concerned with ‘states of denial’ in society about cruel wrongdoing. In relation to CSA he pointed out the ‘passive bystander effect’ of complicit observers and the extent of ‘moral stupor’ and ‘chilling denial’ about child abuse and other cruel expressions of oppressive power in wider society (Cohen 2001). Despite this withdrawal of support from a key leader in the moral panic movement, its advocates persist today.

The rate of CSA has increased with online offending: the internet has been a ‘game changer’. Indecent images of children are sold online, some of which involve in-vivo interactive involvement by the purchaser. Sex offenders posing as peers to children induce them into sexual displays and even personal meetings. The international dimension is not just in relation to trading of abuse online, it also includes the normalisation of child brides, which the UN suggests is the most prevalent version of CSA, a topic we return to in Chapter 8.

Moving to mental health impact, the moral panic claim makers minimised this in terms of scale and individual symptoms. However this is what is known empirically. CSA is linked to educational impairment in child victims. It leads to an over-representation in psychiatric populations and that trend is true of all diagnostic groups, including psychosis.

Moreover, there is a physical health impact. Child victims may suffer anal bleeding and girls, vaginal-vesicular fistulas, affecting their later sex life and reproductive abilities. Adult survivors report other chronic conditions (such as inflammatory bowel disease) so the physical risks are not limited to childhood itself but are lifelong. Apart from this evidence about the psychological and physical impact of the sexual victimisation of children, the implications for psychiatry remain controversial.

For example, mental health assessments *should* ask about childhood adversity, including abuse but in practice this does not typically happen. That evasion might be because of the distraction and false spotlight of the 'present mental state examination' in turn linked to the need to offer a point diagnosis and this displaces the importance of unique biographical formulations. Another point of contention was reflected in the criticisms made during the revision of the Diagnostic and Statistical Manual of the American Psychiatric Association. Some trauma-informed psychiatrists insisted that the term 'borderline personality disorder' (BPD) should be dropped in favour of 'chronic PTSD'.

BPD is defined by the presence of a range of distressed and troublesome conduct. It includes suicidality, self-harm, dramatic panic about the loss of intimates, unstable mood, substance misuse and chaotic social functioning. As with PTSD, it is a fairly capacious concept invented because patients were seen as being on the borderline between neurosis and madness. Whilst the concept is open to question and is constantly disputed by both patients and professionals, the symptoms it subsumes are real enough. The matter of sex differences is important. If chronic PTSD should redefine the predominantly female diagnosis of BPD, then what of men? Combatant PTSD is suffered mainly by men, some of whom become violent, which is rarely seen in females with a diagnosis of BPD. However, the latter diagnosis is common in female prisoners.

PTSD is a unique diagnosis. All of the other functional diagnoses (schizophrenia, depression etc.) by definition have no definable or known etiological origin (that is why they are called 'functional'). However that is not the case with PTSD, indeed a defining feature has to be that there is a recorded history of a traumatic event in the patient's history. The diagnosis of BPD has been the particular focus of feminist critics who note its over-representation in women in a way that might deflect attention from girls being the main victims of sexual predation (Shaw and Proctor 2005).

Whilst these sorts of feminist objections are warranted, they do not exhaust our understanding of the long-term mental health impact of the trauma of CSA, including for boys and men. What is striking from the epidemiological evidence is that CSA predicts over-representation in *all* diagnostic groups, not just BPD, suggesting that CSA has a blunderbuss disruptive effect on a secure sense of self (Read et al. 2003; Varese et al. 2012).

The population labelled with BPD or chronic PTSD reflect inequalities in two senses. First, some people in society live with a history of trauma, whereas others do not. Second, those victims of trauma disproportionately enter the patient role, particularly but not only as psychiatric cases, as it is also linked to chronic physical conditions as well (Lundqvist et al. 2004; Cutajar et al. 2010).

Traditional approaches to examining the link between social group membership (being poor or black or a woman) make visible the likely source of health inequalities (they are named 'dependent variables' or 'social group membership' in research and 'protected characteristics' in some forms of public policy). What the CSA research indicates (and this point applies to survivors of other forms of trauma, falling short of being labelled as PTSD) is that they are an invisible social group, lacking the research recognition of larger clunky groupings, which are taken for granted in social science research.

Survivors of sexual abuse occasionally 'come out' and campaign, but the majority are lost from sight in the interstices of mental health services, living on the streets or in family settings holding dark secrets in the present or from the past. In those places, the historical disclosures of what remain crimes against children may be absent or kept as secrets, amongst just a few relatives and friends. For most victims, historical injustices against them are not recognised and justice passes them by, with their victimiser either dead or living with or without memory or conscience.

For this claim about invisibility to be sustained we need to examine the evidence of the incidence and prevalence of CSA, as well as that related to those with a psychiatric diagnosis. As was argued above such evidence now exists and it is unambiguously damning of a society-wide tendency to minimise the occurrence and implications of CSA. Collectively adults, whether or not they are perpetrators, are to various degrees complicit in this silence about the betrayal of children.

Given the over-representation of survivors of trauma (including, but not only from, CSA) in psychiatric populations, the latter have to contend with further challenges. One is social exclusion, which is an aggravating factor in the unequal treatment and experience of trauma survivors. Psychiatric patients sometimes call themselves 'survivors', which might be a valid self-ascription for a range of reasons. Not only might they have survived CSA and other forms of adversity in childhood, they also have survived coercive detention, the impact of forced treatment and the stigmatisation and distrust of non-patients in wider society. This is a cue for the next section.

Experiencing lost or blocked citizenship: living with a psychiatric diagnosis

The class gradient in psychiatric diagnosis is well established. With the exception of a few diagnostic groupings (anorexia, obsessive-compulsive disorder and bipolar disorder are examples) most neurotic and psychotic symptoms are more prevalent in poorer people. Moreover, as a subgroup of the poor, psychiatric patients encounter further inequalities peculiar to their social positioning in a range of ways. They are disadvantaged in the labour market, which then over-determines a state of chronic poverty and welfare dependence. They are distrusted and stigmatised by others and this often leads to them being socially isolated or relating more comfortably to other patients.

But the most important iniquity suffered is that of state-endorsed and enforced legal discrimination. The state removes liberty without trial, with no guarantee of cure or optimal benign care in return (in ethico-legal terms this is called the 'principle of reciprocity') (Eastman 1994). With the exception of those held under terrorism legislation, no other group in liberal democracies is held recurrently and casually without the protection of a trial, or an advocate for their freedom.

'Mental health law' primarily is not about the enhancement of mental health but the social control of rule transgression. It protects those who are sane by common consent from disruption and anxiety in their daily living. It also protects agents of the state (mental health professionals) from being accused of false imprisonment and assault. Its consequences for identified patients are variable but often negative. It removes them from their daily constraints and opportunities in open society. Forced detention may be traumatic and imposed treatments may be iatrogenic (meaning they cause new harm to the recipient). Psychiatric drugs are life-diminishing and sometimes life-threatening (Brown and Funk 1986; Healy 1997; Kellam 1987).

The consequences of this exclusion in the nineteenth and the bulk of the twentieth century were the 'warehousing' of madness, out of sight and out of mind. The social administrative challenge of madness became evident with the emergence of the workhouse system. Its managers became aware that most paupers complied with daily expectations of labour and institutional routines. However, lunatics defied these expectations, setting the scene for the more specialist asylum system.

During the late twentieth century in Western democracies, the social administrative norm of the asylum system was opposed for a variety of reasons. These large hospitals were expensive and so 'decarceration' offered a fiscal advantage to the state. Also, user critics and dissenting professionals attacked the dehumanising routines of 'total institutions' and their iatrogenic impact on psychological functioning, well known since the 1960s (Sedgwick 1982).

The demolition of the old large hospitals did not alter though the continuing role of smaller acute psychiatric units, aimed at the daily detention and forced treatment of patients. Mental health law went on undiminished, with these units very rarely now recording the voluntary status of their residents. Even when that rarity is recorded, it may reflect a pseudo-voluntary status (Szmukler and Appelbaum 2008). The existence of powers of coercion makes true voluntarism from patients difficult to discern and record validly. Moreover, inpatient legal control was merely extended to community settings, with ensured drugging leading to a sort of 'tranquil prison' in the patient's home (Fabris 2011; Rugkåsa 2016).

Given these unresolved concerns about human rights, on the one hand there was an international consensus that such controls were a sign of social progress (to ensure patients in need were treated) but, on the other, there was a counter-discourse that such powers were discriminatory and oppressive. Indeed some reports from the UN about mental health services and torture pointed out an overlap in cruel and degrading treatment in the two forms of state intervention (Pūrasis 2017). Mental health services were and remain a controversial focus about *denied personal recognition*, as discussed earlier by Axel Honneth. Such services try, often in vain, to be 'both kindly and efficacious' to use a criterion set by Sedgwick (ibid) and revisited by Pilgrim (2018b).

The users' movement and 'Mad Studies'

Given these persistent and unresolved human rights questions, woven into coercive mental health work, the service users' movement (sometimes called 'ex-patients', 'survivors' or 'consumer' movement) emerged in the 1970s, on the back of more established New Social Movements established a decade earlier (Crossley 2006).

Debates about the opposition to the very existence of mental health law also remained, in both radical user and professional arenas. Complaints that authoritarian regimes, such as the case of psychiatric detention of political dissidents in the Soviet Union, were misusing medicine raised the question about why its *use* in routine psychiatric practice in the West was acceptable in principle (Cohen 1989; Bloch and Reddaway 1977).

One outcrop of this unresolved contention about impaired citizenship was the self-organised intellectual work of radicalised patients. They formed study groups about their personal and collective history and even proudly established the academic project of 'Mad Studies', which emerged from what can be called 'organic intellectuals' (Russo and Sweeney 2016).

Although genuine attempts at rescuing the damaged citizenship of psychiatric patients have been evident, especially in relation to both anti-stigma campaigns and the 'recovery movement', a caution remains about such optimistic policy aspirations and despite recovery rhetoric the structural obstacle of coercion and its human rights implications remain.

Even if legalism were to be abandoned (and a legitimate political and ethical justification exists for this desire), a deeply instilled cultural fear of madness would still be there. Mad people over time and place have never had an easy time. Chained, rejected, mocked, detained and drugged, the ready justifications for their ill treatment are ingrained. There is little wonder that in the public imagination the problem with legalism is that it may culminate in 'wrongful detention' (implying illogically that 'rightful' detention is morally acceptable for its recipients). This common fear suggests that most of us know that any offers from agents of the state for 'the treatment of mental illness', will probably be neither desirable nor life enhancing. Few of us queue up for a diagnosis of 'major mental illness' that might culminate in detentions without trial.

Madness emerges and is labelled in ordinary settings, *before* doctors codify with their rubber-stamping diagnoses, or agents of the state do their best or worst (Coulter 1973). The overarching position of 'the social', within the biopsychosocial model we discussed earlier, is relevant to this caution about the restored citizenship for psychiatric patients.

There is a large hill to climb if those entering the psychiatric system are to have their unequal social status reversed or their rule transgressions tolerated. One reason for this is not only the latter social reaction to difference, once a psychiatric patient's career develops and becomes visible in their conduct in open systems (e.g., talking to their voices). There is also a primary concern for the *original* loss of reason, if this is known to friends, neighbours employers etc., even if the person is no longer symptomatic.

We lose our reason at our peril, if the word gets out. A 'known history of mental illness' is a calling card few of us enjoy carrying (Pescosolido et al. 2013; Angermeyer and Schulze 2001). This led to the advice from David Cooper, the only psychiatrist willing to accept the label of being an 'anti-psychiatrist', that if we are to go mad, then we should try to do so discreetly (Cooper 1968). This of course is difficult to sustain, as mad people tend not to be discreet in their strange actions and speech. As a leading British user activist, Peter Campbell, recently deceased, recalled in conversation a few years ago 'having a diagnosis of schizophrenia has not exactly helped me on the dancefloors of life'; see also, Campbell (1996).

Psychiatric patient-hood emerges in modern societies as a result of those diagnosed failing in their role expectations (in common with physical health problems) but especially because they *unintelligibly* transgress rules. Psychotic patients (the main group now detained in acute mental health services) bear the long-term implications of their loss of reason being linked in the public imagination to a loss of social credibility. With that comes a fear and distrust of patients and ex-patients. We can contrast this with the sympathy readily invoked about depression and anxiety, which are treated in primary care and are rarely linked to involvement with statutory mental health services. Because they are 'common' mental disorders, and fear and sadness are readily understood emotions, they invoke compassion. By contrast being unintelligible is different; those sane by common consent are frightened when mad conduct emerges in their midst. Accordingly, to lose one's reason risks being cast in the role of someone to be permanently distrusted, which makes citizenship precarious.

Psychotic patients break a fundamental duty, noted above, of adult humans to be socially intelligible, when and if required. The silent but implicitly known meta-rule, which we learn during our primary socialisation, is that we must account for ourselves, as we mature into adulthood. When required, we must display intelligibility about, and take responsibility for, our actions. The added transgression of this meta-rule may leave a sense of distrust about the insane (recovered or not), from those who are sane by common consent and have never personally received a psychiatric diagnosis.

Those committed to 'Mad Studies' recognise this long-term struggle (Castrodale 2015). At times this recognition extends to resisting attempts to be re-socialised or brought back into the fold of society. The latter pressure can be traced back to moral treatment in the nineteenth century. Today mental health work still has rule enforcement as its central goal. Those chronically or episodically battling against those efforts (i.e. patients coerced into compliance) may at times wish to celebrate, rather than recover from, madness ('mad pride').

That subgroup of patients resent and refuse to be ashamed of their non-conformity. Their political strategy might then extend to survivors taking on a permanent identity, shared with other patients. What for medicine might be a description of 'severe and enduring mental illness' might for those in Mad Studies and the 'anti-recovery movement', be a positive attempt at new forms of identity formation and group solidarity.

Thus a push back from some survivor groups is now apparent. They demand the right *not* to recover, on the grounds that their experiences warrant a legitimate life outside of the expectations of normality (Fromm's 'pathology of normalcy') and without the oppression of psychiatric interference. Instead they prefer to focus on their creativity and their authentic insights by defying social conformity. They dismiss the 'recovery star' (a pictorial measure of dimensions of clinical and social improvement) as a 'recovery crucifix', because it doubly stigmatises those who are unable or unwilling to abandon their mad way of being. Their campaigns then extend not just to the right to be 'unrecovered', but also to finding points of solidarity with other chronically impoverished groups in society. However, given that conformity and the meta-rule of social intelligibility ipso facto define normativity in all human societies, the prospects for the routine social tolerance of 'unrecovered' psychiatric patients for now are poor.

Conclusion

This chapter has considered the matter of living with inequality by focusing on the relationship between normal alienation and psychological abnormality. Normal alienation considered by Sennett, Frankfurt School members and others, and traceable to Marx and Freud, is driven by psychosocial forces that also are relevant to the unfortunate traumatic lives of some, but not others, in our midst. Some of those go on to enter the world of psychiatric patienthood, where more attacks on their self-esteem and dignity, and constraints on their citizenship, await. One psychosocial insult is added to another, as the casualties of deliberate violence and accidental shock are shepherded into deeper dysfunctional states of existence and social marginalisation.

The precarious boundary between normal alienation and psychological abnormality is not merely a matter of semantics, though how we conceptualise it is more or less helpful, depending on our contingent role(s) in life. These epistemological concerns are also responding to ontological ones. Fear and sadness are real and are manifested routinely in a range of physiological and cognitive indicators of distress in response to actual threats, in all mammals, not just humans. We can all recognise our frightened or unhappy pet dog. Madness and incorrigibility lack the same biological and behavioural tangibility but their implications for the flow of daily life are very real for identified patients and those who are sane by common consent. They reflect problems across all societies because normativity and a sensibility about rules and their transgression exist in all open human systems.

Psychological dysfunction is a social judgment but in its own way still real. Little or no training is required to describe it in a context in which are all socialised. We have moral expectations about ourselves and others about rule compliance and role competence. We can be troubled and troubling and sometimes both. Those who are distressed, unintelligible or incorrigible struggle to comply with rules, in whole or part because their own personhood has not been respected or recognised. Their deviance often then triggers a vicious circle of further social invalidation and social defeat.

The way those psychosocial processes are played out, in what Szasz preferred to call 'problems of living', invites our serious reflection. He opted to re-frame the conventional description of mental illness as being about the gaming of interpersonal power (with winners and losers), not the self-evident jurisdiction of medicine. Our view is that a more complex and uncertain open system exists but in which moral agency (emphasised by Szasz) is certainly in play. That complexity includes the uneven conditions of possibility in society for people to conform to expectations of being rational and rule compliant. Some of us are in a better position than others to come up to scratch in this regard, as the evidence on adverse childhood events is now making clear.

Returning to the graffiti we started with: the 'horrible' period between birth and death is more painful for some of us than others. Inequality remains a hallmark of human life, not just the common experience of suffering. In the next chapter this point is extended and illustrated further.

References

Babiak, P., and R.D. Hare. 2007. *Snakes in Suits: When Psychopaths Go to Work*. New York: Harper Collins.

Angermeyer, M.C., and B. Schulze. 2001. "Reinforcing Stereotypes: How the Focus on Forensic Cases in News Reporting May Influence Public Attitudes Towards the Mentally Ill." *International Journal of Law and Psychiatry* 24 (5): 469–486.

Bateson, G. 1980. *Mind and Nature: A Necessary Unity*. New York: Bantam Books.

Berrios, G.E. 1988. "Obsessional Disorders During the Nineteenth Century: Terminological and Classificatory Issues." In *The Anatomy of Madness* (vol. 1), edited by W.F. Bynum, R. Porter, and M. Shepherd, 55–67. London: Tavistock.

Bezo, B., and S. Maggi. 2015. "Living in 'Survival Mode:' Intergenerational Transmission of Trauma from the Holodomor Genocide of 1932–1933 in Ukraine." *Social Science and Medicine* 134: 87–94.

Bhaskar, R. 2008. *Dialectic: The Pulse of Freedom*. London: Routledge.

Bloch, S., and P. Reddaway. 1977. *Russia's Political Hospitals: The Abuse of Psychiatry in the Soviet Union*. London: Viktor Gollanz.

Bowlby, J. 1951. *Maternal Care and Mental Health*. Geneva: World Health Organization.

Brown, P., and S.C. Funk. 1986. "Tardive Dyskinesia: Barriers to the Professional Recognition of Iatrogenic Disease." *Journal of Health and Social Behavior* 27: 116–132.

Campbell, P. 1996. "The History of the User Movement in the United Kingdom." In *Mental Health Matters: A Reader*, edited by T. Heller, J. Reynolds, R. Gomm, R. Muston, and S. Pattison, 67–80. Buckingham: Open University Press.

Castrodale, M.A. 2015. "Mad Matters: A Critical Reader in Canadian Mad Studies." *Scandinavian Journal of Disability Research* 17 (3): 284–246.

Children's Commissioner's Report. 2016. *Barnahus: Improving the Response to Child Sexual Abuse in England*. London: UK Children's Commissioner's Office.

Cohen, D. 1989. *Soviet Psychiatry*. London: Paladin.

Cohen, S. 2001. *States of Denial: Knowing About Atrocities and Suffering*. Cambridge: Polity.

Cohen, S., and L. Taylor. 1992. *Escape Attempts: The Theory and Practice of Resistance to Everyday Life*. London: Routledge.

Cooper, D. 1968. *Psychiatry and Anti-psychiatry*. London: Tavistock.

Coulter, J. 1973. *Approaches to Insanity*. New York: Wiley.

Crossley, N. 2006. *Contesting Psychiatry: Social Movements in Mental Health*. London: Routledge.

Cutajar, M.C., P.E. Mullen, J.R.P. Ogloff, S.D. Thomas, D.L. Wells, and J. Spataro. 2010. "Psychopathology in a Large Cohort of Sexually Abused Children Followed up to 43 Years." *Child Abuse and Neglect* 34 (11): 813–822.

Eastman, N. 1994. "Mental Health Law: Civil Liberties and the Principle of Reciprocity." *British Medical Journal* 308: 43.

Engel, G.L. 1980. "The Clinical Application of the Biopsychosocial Model." *American Journal of Psychiatry* 137: 535–544.

Fabris, E. 2011. *Tranquil Prisons: Chemical Incarceration Under Community Treatment Orders*. Toronto: University of Toronto Press.

Fish, F. 1968. *Clinical Psychopathology*. Bristol: John Wright.

Fowler, J.H., and N.A. Christakis. 2008. "The Dynamic Spread of Happiness in a Large Social Network: Longitudinal Analysis Over 20 Years in the Framingham Heart Study." *British Medical Journal* 337: a2338.

Fraser, N. (1997). *Justice Interruptus: Critical Reflections on the 'Postsocialist' Condition*. New York and London: Routledge.

Freud, S. 1930. *Civilisation and Its Discontents*. London: Hogarth Press.

Fromm, E. 1944. "Individual and Social Origins of Neurosis." *American Sociological Review* 4 (4): 10–15.

Fromm, E. 1955. *The Sane Society*. New York: Holt, Rinehart and Winston.

Habermas, J. 1989. "The Tasks of a Critical Theory of Society." In *Critical Theory and Society: A Reader*, edited by S.E. Bronner and D.M. Kellner, 12–24. London: Routledge.

Healy, D. 1997. *The Anti-Depressant Era*. London: Harvard University Press.

Honneth, A. 2007. *Disrespect: The Normative Foundations of Critical Theory*. Cambridge: Polity Press.

Horkheimer, M. 1931. "Die Gegenwärtige Lage der Sozialphilosophie und die Aufgaben eines Instituts für Sozialforschung." *Frankfurter Universitätsreden* 37: 13–20.

Horwitz, A., and J. Wakefield. 2007. *The Loss of Sadness: How Psychiatry Transformed Normal Sorrow into Depressive Disorder*. New York: Oxford University Press.

Johnstone, L. and M. Boyle with J. Cromby, J. Dillon, D. Harper, P. Kinderman, E. Longden, D. Pilgrim, and J. Read. 2018. *The Power Threat Meaning Framework: Towards the Identification of Patterns in Emotional Distress, Unusual Experiences and Troubled or Troubling Behaviour*. Leicester: British Psychological Society.

Kellam, A.M.P. 1987. "The Neuroleptic Syndrome, So Called: A Survey of the World Literature." *British Journal of Psychiatry* 150: 752–759.

Lane, C. 2008. *Shyness: How Normal Behavior Became a Sickness*. New Haven: Yale University Press.

Lundqvist, G., K. Hansson, and C.G. Svedin. 2004. "The Influence of Childhood Sexual Abuse Factors on Women's Health." *Nordic Journal of Psychiatry* 58 (5): 395–401.

Masson, J. 1985. *The Assault on Truth: Freud's Suppression of the Seduction Theory*. Harmondsworth: Penguin.

May, P.A., C.D. Chambers, W.O. Kalberg, et al. February 2018. "Prevalence of Fetal Alcohol Spectrum Disorders in 4 US Communities." *JAMA* 319 (5): 474–482. doi:10.1001/jama.2017.21896.

Pescosolido, B.A., T.R. Medina, J.K. Martin, and J.S. Long. 2013. "The 'Backbone' of Stigma: Identifying the Global Core of Public Prejudice Associated with Mental Illness." *American Journal of Public Health* 103 (5): 853–860.

Pilgrim, D. 2018a. *Child Sexual Abuse: Moral Panic or State of Denial?* London: Routledge.

Pilgrim, D. 2018b. "Are Kindly and Efficacious Mental Health Services Possible?" *Journal of Mental Health* 27 (4): 295–297.

Pilgrim, D. 2015. "The Biopsychosocial Model in Health Research: Its' Strength and Limitations for Critical Realists." *Journal of Critical Realism* 14 (2): 164–180.

Pilgrim, D., A. Rogers, and R.P. Bentall. 2009. "The Centrality of Personal Relationships in the Creation and Amelioration of Mental Health Problems: The Current Interdisciplinary Case." *Health* 13: 235–254.

Pūrasis, D. 2017. *Report of the Special Rapporteur on the Right of Everyone to the Enjoyment of the Highest Attainable Standard of Physical and Mental Health*. Geneva: UN Human Rights Council.

Read, J., K. Agar, N. Argyle, and V. Aderhold. 2003. "Sexual and Physical Abuse during Childhood as Predictors of Hallucinations, Delusions and Thought Disorder." *Psychology and Psychotherapy* 76 (1): 1–22.

Ross, E.J., D.L. Graham, K.M. Money, and G.D. Stanwood. 2015. "Developmental Consequences of Fetal Exposure to Drugs: What We Know and What We Still Must Learn." *Neuropsychopharmacology* 40 (1): 61–87.

Rugkåsa, J. 2016. "Effectiveness of Community Treatment Orders: The International Evidence." *Canadian Journal of Psychiatry* 61: 15–24.

Russo, J., and A. Sweeney, eds. 2016. *Searching for a Rose Garden: Challenging Psychiatry, Fostering Mad Studies*. Monmouth: PCCS Books.

Scheff, T. 1966. *Being Mentally Ill: A Sociological Theory*. Chicago: Aldine.

Sedgwick, P. 1982. *Psychopolitics*. London: Pluto Press.

Sennett, R. 2003. *Respect: The Formation of Character in an Age of Inequality*. London: Penguin.

Sennett, R., and J. Cobb. 1972. *The Hidden Injuries of Class*. New York: Vintage.

Shaw, C., and G. Proctor. 2005. "I. Women at the Margins: A Critique of the Diagnosis of Borderline Personality Disorder." *Feminism and Psychology* 15 (4): 483–490.

Shephard, B. 2002. *A War on Nerves: Soldiers and Psychiatrists 1914-1994*. London: Pimlico.

Steptoe, A., E.L. Gibson, M. Hamer, and J. Wardle. 2007. "Neuroendocrine and Cardiovascular Correlates of Positive Affect Measure by Ecological Momentary Assessment and by Questionnaire." *Psychoneuroendocrininology* 32 (1): 56–64.

Szasz, T.S. 1961. "The Uses of Naming and the Origin of the Myth of Mental Illness." *American Psychologist* 16: 59–65.

Szmukler, G., and P. Appelbaum. 2001. "Treatment Pressures, Coercion and Compulsion." In *Textbook of Community Psychiatry*, edited by G. Thornicroft and G. Szmukler. Oxford: Oxford University Press.

Szmukler, G., and P. S. Appelbaum. 2008. Treatment pressures, leverage, coercion, and compulsion in mental health care. *Journal of Mental Health, 17*(3): 233–244.

Varese, F., F. Smeets, M. Drukker, et al. 2012. "Childhood Adversities Increase the Risk of Psychosis: A Meta-analysis of Patient-Control, Prospective and Cross-Sectional Cohort Studies." *Schizophrenia Bulletin* 38 (4): 661–671.

8 Tired of living and scared of dying

Introduction

The previous chapter looked at the notion, and the uneven distribution, of suffering. This chapter extends that discussion, with examples of existential challenges that we might encounter between birth and death, depending on who we are and where we are at a moment in time. It allows us to consider a matter that we introduce in the next and earlier chapters – intersectionality and social group membership. The dimensions reported in mainstream social epidemiology and medical sociology, and reflected in our work on mental health and illness include social class ('socio-economic status'), sex (or 'gender'), race and ethnicity, age, sexuality and disability (Rogers and Pilgrim 2020). If these are investigated singularly, then evidence shaped by those categories alone will miss the complexity of their multiple interactions.

Intersectionality brings together synergies, which create particular average risks or benefits to well-being and wealth to those in overlapping social groups. Later, that initial conceptual emphasis of *social causation*, referring to trends in *groups*, shifted more to a kaleidoscope of *identities* and multiple versions of the experience of oppression for *individuals*. For this reason, the meaning of 'intersectionality' is worth clarifying in the literature which uses it. With that conceptual distinction in mind, the two complementary versions of 'intersectionality' are useful to consider, because they help to illuminate complexity. If inequalities are *both* multiple antecedents (activated causes rooted in socio-economic, sexual and racial divisions) *and* they lead to a multiplicity of experienced personal outcomes, then we can try to make sense of that complexity. Alongside this keeping all three balls in the air of the biological, the psychological and the social, any analysis can be challenging because in the literature at times the emphasis is on extrinsic causes but at other times is on the experience of multiply-disadvantaged people. Both reflect a connotation of 'intersectionality'.

As the title of this chapter suggests, we are all in our own ways, and to various degrees, tired of living and scared of dying. What is of interest here are variations on this theme during the life span. The privileging of socio-economic determinants (especially social class) as we noted in the previous chapters requires caveats about contradictions and exceptional cases, within

DOI: 10.4324/9781003025641-8

overall trends. If our focus is on the lifespan, we find that the highest rates of mental health problems are in the very young and the very old.

Time ensures shifts in existential security in a range of ways for individuals, but it also is a characteristic of the systems they are embedded within, which are subject to changing quickly or slowly. Place or 'locale' is another pathway into understanding variations in experience. An obvious example of this is reflected in the use of resources by those who have them to buy property in places seen to be propitious for their health (leafy suburbs, quiet villages and seaside idylls). Poorer people have little or no such choice. Over time people want choices about where and how they age in places they prefer and feel secure. Ageing in a chosen place has advantages. These include a sense of attachment and connection to a familiar location, feelings of security in relation to home, supportive local communities and a linking sense of identity with known surroundings (Wiles et al. 2021). These expectations become more relevant in older age, because home rather than work becomes the focus of daily living.

As we proceed from birth to death and encounter and resolve (or not), recurring existential challenges, different age periods are relevant to note. A psychoanalytical revisionist Erik Erikson offered a social psychological model of this personal journey. He suggested seven main stages: (1) trust versus mistrust (early infancy); (2) autonomy versus shame ('potty training'); (3) initiative versus guilt (pre-school exploration); (4) industry versus inferiority (schooling adjustment); (5) identity versus role confusion (peer relationships in adolescence); (6) intimacy versus isolation (sexual intimacy); (7) generativity versus stagnation (work life and parenting); and (8) ego integrity versus despair (reflections on life). In this chapter our focus is on phases 5 and 7 whilst doing our best to consider the biological, psychological and social aspects of living through the life span.

Tired of living and scared of growing up during adolescence

The periodisation offered by Erikson is rough and ready and the caveat of longer history has to be addressed. Adolescence is both a social construct and has an anchor point in biological reality. In some parts of the world the permitted age of marriage is low or non-existent. Some states in the USA still permit very young brides. When the latter are pre-pubescent they are at physical risk of genital injury and, after puberty, they are at risk of birth complications, if they become pregnant. In addition social impairments accrue: the child bride is typically no longer schooled but is placed in a domestic role and they lose their peer relationships for age. Dubious sexual and patriarchal ideologies have been used to depict children as being just small adults 'participating' in sexual contact with the elders, which evades any consideration of uneven discrepancies of power and cognitive capacity during the life span. Women married after the age of 18 years have been found to be more involved in household decision-making processes than child-brides, whereas child-brides were more likely to experience various forms of spousal abuse and violence in married life (Abera et al. 2020). If a person reaches adolescence having been in a war zone or the victim of child sexual abuse, then their maturation and self-confidence will *already* be damaged, which could affect the existential challenges of adolescence.

The period of adolescence is relevant for dealing with identity formation. In recent times, this has been reflected in the controversies surrounding gender non-conforming youngsters (Brunskell-Evans and Moore 2018; Cohen and Barnes 2019). This inner challenge of leaving childhood to become a self-possessed adult is not only a personal one but it co-occurs with the interpersonal context of judgement made by older generations. Subcultural definitions of an emerging generation surface at times through rebellion and transgression.

Studies of moral panics after the Second World War (Cohen 1972; Young 1971) focused upon teenage male gangs in violent conflict ('Mods and Rockers'). Other groups of teenagers included illicit drug users and the so-called 'aggressive' girl gangs. Most moral panics reflect a negative attribution about identifiable subgroups of young poor people (an exception here is paedophiles, who are older and come from all class backgrounds, including elite groups). The main behavioural focus of these young groups is on risky conduct, which impacts negatively on the well-being of others, but also puts perpetrators at risk from violence or drug abuse.

Not all moral panics have been linked to young people, but the majority have, which reminds us that Erikson's identity formation brings with it interpersonal (social cognitive) processes, and so the intergenerational field becomes important to consider. This is a social, not just a psychological, matter. Erikson's schema of the life span challenges assumed that failure in an early stage of development affects the likely success of subsequent ones, as time passes. Developmental failure in childhood can trigger later psychological regression, with new life events or periods of adjustment such as adolescence. That point about the risk of regression to weak points from the past is pertinent when we now address an eating disorder, which is particularly associated with adolescence.

Anorexia nervosa and adolescence

When faced with the imminent prospect of growing up, which the bodily signs of puberty signal to the child, this poses psychological not just physical challenges. Much is made often about the psychological impact of hormone surges. However, the adolescent also has more to cope with than this: adulthood beckons (or threatens) with its prospects for work and sex. Easing away from adult authority domestically and in school settings helps that transition and is negotiated more or less politely by teenagers. They become peer-orientated to establish their position as, and within, a new generation. Sometimes they are wayward and boundary testing, at others they are compliant with the expectations of their elders.

Given this general process of existential transition, why do some adolescents starve themselves and why are most of them girls? Also, why do they believe that they are fat when they are in fact thin? Two initial observations when answering these questions are that Erikson noted possible earlier developmental failures, and feminists have highlighted the uneven contemporary pressure on girls more than boys to be body conscious (Elks 1994; Marcotte et al. 2002; Parker and Mauger 1976; Blowers et al. 2003).

As this phase, quickly approaching the next one of early adulthood, has an existential focus on *identity* then the imagined world of being a mature adult, on the close horizon of time is important. Identity uncertainty and exploration are normal in teenage years. However, this process is more challenging for some than others. The physical presentation of body shape and its sexual signalling, physiological changes and the potential for child bearing, are common points of reflection for teenage girls. Food and its over- or under-consumption can be a ready focus for control over the body. Body image can become a preoccupation in adolescence and may continue well into adulthood. That trend can be seen in those who are prone to anorexia (athletes, dancers and models) and applies to young men as well as women, though less often (Drewnowski et al. 1995).

This picture invites us to apply a biopsychosocial explanation for anorexia. For example, starvation when encountered or imposed on non-anorexic subjects seems to increase the risk of depressed appetite. That is, if we are starved, when food then becomes available we are less likely to return to previous levels of appetite and food consumption. (There may be a neurochemical effect operating here to depress appetite, once starvation appears.)

In areas of the world with low incomes and disrupted food supplies, because of drought or poverty, the incidence of anorexia in low but the general population tends to be slimmer than in Western societies. (This is a reminder that the complementary risk to the health of children in the West is obesity – see Chapter 3.)

The case of South Africa is illustrative; here the prevalence of anorexia is nearly as high as in the US or Europe, whereas it is low in the rest of sub-Saharan Africa. South Africa is the richest country in the region and so the prevalence of anorexia (and obesity) seems to be driven by system-wide relative affluence, which has direct and indirect aspects. The direct commercial point is the availability and promotion of obesogenic foodstuffs, and the indirect cultural impact is that body shape is also commodified, especially but not only for females. Anorexia, and the diet and fashion industry, are part of this interaction of economic drivers and cultural pressures, especially on young women.

Notwithstanding this context we still need to understand why not *all* adolescents suffer from anorexia; they represent a subgroup, and yet the whole group is subject to the commercial and cultural forces just noted. The estimates vary of incidence and prevalence across space. Apart from richer countries having higher rates, there are also within-country differences. For example in the Netherlands there are no regional differences in incidence for anorexia but bulimia (gorging and vomiting) is higher in city dwellers. The incidence of anorexia has been steady since the 1970s, though over time the tendency was for the condition to be reported in younger children (Smink et al. 2012).

Taken together, lifetime prevalence studies in Western countries tell us that anorexia is higher in women (around 4%) but only around 0.3% in men. Whilst this sex difference is significant its overall prevalence is still low (i.e., 96% of females never become anorexic) and points to the need to account for particular biopsychosocial characteristics of young anorexics in more detail. The average age of onset in the life span is 18 years and that reflects a distribution back to childhood (Volpe et al. 2016). It also is a broad indicator that the cusp between adolescence and young adulthood is an important existential transitional point, with a peak of incidence then.

There is some evidence that there may be a genetic bias, but none to indicate that it is a female-only phenomenon. If girls are more, but not uniquely, vulnerable, compared to boys, then genetics offers us no persuasive singular explanation. The genetic hypothesis is supported by low incidence levels world-wide, with no country being completely free of self-starving young people, but undermined by both sex differences and regional differences. Self-starvation as a form of *political defiance* is a common phenomenon (hunger-striking), which might be pertinent to understanding anorexia (Orbach 1986). The case of anorexia could be re-framed as a sort of micro-civil war, with those lacking power (actual and perceived) resisting the more powerful. The anorexic young person is displaying a particular form of control in relation to others and possibly in relation to impeding the existential shift from childhood to adulthood.

As far as class is concerned, this is an outlier, compared to other forms of psychological abnormality, because it is more likely in middle-class girls. Sometimes eating disorders are de-medicalised and euphemised as 'eating distress'. However, with the close comparator of hunger-striking in mind, who is distressed? Is it the thin child claiming that she is fat or is it her parent fearing, quite understandably, that she may die? 'Distress' in this case is part of an interpersonal field rather than residing in one person.

Answering the question of sex differences under the cultural pressures of affluent societies returns us in part to sexed cultural messages in the mass media and invites feminist critiques. When accounting for anorexia being a minority of young people interactionist explanations are suggested. In individual cases we do not know for certain the particular origins of anorexia as self-starvation accompanied by a distorted body image.

Psychologically, anorexia is linked to obsessive cognitive styles: patients with anorexia tend to be perfectionistic. It is more common, in higher-achieving youngsters, who may excel scholastically or in the arts or sport. The determination to control – *both* to achieve *and* to focus on food and weight, are a shared personality capability. These are clues or trends but not definitive answers about individual cases.

Anorexia is a version of defiance to the norms of conformity but with a price to be paid. It includes osteoporosis and proneness to fractures, cardiac pathology, anaemia, amenorrhea in females and low testosterone in males, electrolyte abnormalities and kidney pathology and sudden death. As far as the last on the list is concerned, this includes suicide and complications from the list of raised pathology. Anorexia then is a serious life-threatening condition, at the very point in the life span when death is least expected.

Prolonged starvation at some point will probably end in premature death, though sustained moderately low levels of food intake might be linked to *longer* life expectancy, i.e., lean people, on average, live longer than fat people (Samaras et al. 2002). And a caveat here is that frail older people sometimes develop very late onset anorexia, as appetite declines with age and depression increases, and consequently they may become both underweight and malnourished (Wysokiński et al. 2005).

Even if we never know, with certainty, why some individual youngsters starve themselves and others do not, some themes of explanation do recur in the literature. For example, anorexic young people do have a tendency towards perfectionism in their habits and a need to feel in control (Lloyd et al. 2014). Other general conditions of possibility, which increase the risk of anorexia seem to be living in an affluent society; the shaping role of mass media in relation to sexed body image; the role of social media in sustaining anorexic behaviour; the use of food as an instrument of both personal and interpersonal control; and finally the existential fear of impending adulthood. On the last note, the starving young woman or man defies growing into being an adult, both as an internal experience and external display.

As Erikson noted, the chances of successfully resolving the tensions in a particular life stage, rely in part, on the confidence bequeathed from earlier phases. For this reason, any formulation in the clinic of a *particular* case, could take that (biopsychosocial) point in mind. Some of the psychosocial considerations about the development of anorexia in adolescence are also pertinent to the next case study, especially in relation to why identity and its control are an existential matter.

Older age and its existential challenges

To extend the historical caveat we noted above about childhood, older age has a particular and routine meaning in developed countries in modernity. However, in the past the average age of death was what we would now consider to be middle adulthood. Warfare and infectious diseases created a world that was 'short and brutish'. In the Middle Ages the average age of death ranged between 30 and 40 years of age (linked to locality and class position). In Europe life expectancy doubled between the middle of the nineteenth century and today. Infant mortality at first retarded this trend, so those surviving into adulthood reflected more and more on their mortality and the limitations that might accrue in old age.

Existential considerations of impending mortality are today more typically for those who live beyond middle age. It also means that causes of death predominate now that were less common than in the past (such as cancer and dementia) because before the nineteenth century most people did not live long enough to experience these conditions. The twentieth century has seen a shift in societal thinking about old age. For people reaching retirement age there are many competing and contradictory messages about age and ageing well or badly. The absence of linearity between chronological age and bodily fitness and the clear variation in the expression of physical ageing has complicated any simple biological account of human ageing.

Additionally sociological analysis has suggested that much of what we consider to be 'ageing' emerges from social practices. Gilleard and Higgs (2009) have suggested that a 'third age' constituted by people (including at the time of writing 'baby boomers'), who created youth culture five decades ago, are now reaching advanced years. Later life is seen as a lifestyle, which one can participate in to the degree that one wants to and retain a sense of youth culture in everyday life which is actually ageless.

In a more general sense it has been suggested that there has been a shift in the mechanisms of health inequalities in developed countries from the direct effect of capital to class habitus. Living into very old age is also socially patterned. There are stark variations in healthy ageing outcomes and ageing-related health between different social groups. People with higher educational attainment and income, who have had better jobs earlier on in life, tend towards better physical and cognitive functioning, compared to those who have had a lifetime experience of socio-economic disadvantage. The latter are also more likely to develop ill health and die earlier than those who have had more advantages (MacGuire 2020).

Turning to the psychological dimensions of older age and the prospect of impending finitude, humans are unique in imagining and recognising their own death. Erickson, and others such as Carl Jung, viewed the final stage of life as one of meaning seeking and reflection during that recognition of personal mortality. The chances of success rely in part on the degree to which past stages were resolved satisfactorily.

Clearly then a psychological dimension to ageing is important to consider. However, when we examine inequalities in old age both *biological* and *social* factors are important to explain differences in why some of us satisfactorily come to terms with our particular lives and our impending death. Any burden of past psychopathology might be inflected by newly emergent biological and social events in a person's life.

An elephant in the room is that as we get older we are more prone to physical morbidity and are more likely to die (notwithstanding the point made above about baby boomers identifying with youth culture, and this image it creates of being 'forever young'). Chronic physical conditions prior to death may be lived with for many years and for some decades. These bring pain, social impairments and a need to be in regular contact with healthcare professionals. Thus, bio-social interactions become more relevant in old age, than in younger years.

For example, social restriction may reflect the synergies of mobility problems, limited public transport, loss of driving capacity, the relative or absolute loss of sensory acuity, poverty and the loss of social networks. The latter may accrue from loss of work colleagues and from an aggregating loss of friends and family. The longer one lives the more likely that our peers will die. This then increases the prospects of depression, with recurrent mourning experiences, as does living with chronic pain. If care is required for our increasing frailty then the rich will have better prospects than others to buffer the excesses of their declining quality of life.

The socio-economic burden of illness and impairment in old age on younger generations might also shift with demographic changes. If the young have lower birth rates but the old continue to live in large numbers, then responses to the strain of care capability will increase in a population, reflected in both alcohol use and suicide. Socio-economic inequalities in care use and provision place greater emotional and physical burdens on those both giving and receiving care. Having to rely on help provided by families because of a lack of availability of publicly provided services restricts access to formal care more amongst people from lower socio-economic status groups.

Lower-educated individuals and those with household incomes below the national median are more likely to live in a nursing home (Bernardi et al. 2021). Additionally, poorer individuals are less likely to be able to buy formal care on the market than the rich and are thus more likely to rely more on informal care provided by families or on poorer quality nursing home provision. The suggested existence of 'social care deserts' in England in recent years draws attention to the impact of geographical and other inequalities on the availability, quality and experience of residential, nursing and domiciliary care for those living in more deprived situations (Higgs et al. 2022).

Alcohol use in older age

The uneven impact of alcohol on physical and mental health is present from conception. In the previous chapter foetal-alcohol syndrome was noted. If we escape that eventuality (as most of us do), then differential patterns of both the use and the adverse impact of alcohol continue. For example, alcohol consumption is linked to intra-familial abuse and road traffic collision deaths and injury, which can impact on children before they use the substance personally. At the other end of the life span, concerns have been expressed by public health experts in recent times about the deleterious effects of alcohol.

This section addresses this concern and traces its origins and concerns using a biopsychosocial frame of reference. The biological aspects of alcohol use are better known than other chemical substances affecting behaviour and experience, because it has been woven into the development of our species for centuries. Although, with some exceptions of cultures which claim population-wide abstinence for religious reasons, alcohol use is a universal phenomenon.

Over the life stages there are socially determined changes to drinking behaviour. Young single people with healthier livers are more likely to drink heavily and socially. In early middle age, drinking is peer-orientated and accounted for in terms of being in control through continuing with the responsibilities of work and parenting. Later on in middle age, we may develop strategies for neutralising alcohol-related health risks through compensatory strategies of exercise (Emslie et al. 2012). Social networks of drinking then become less diverse and shrink, as we move from middle age to older age (Kim et al. 2016).

Psychologically, the immediate impact of alcohol ingestion is pleasant. It makes people feel relaxed and might increase confidence. Its impact on the whole brain includes the frontal lobes, increasing disinhibition of speech and action. People become more sociable, opinionated and voluble. They drown their sorrows and celebrate successes with the drug. The downside at the individual level is that people may say and do things they later regret. This can extend to reckless, anti-social and illegal acts. Violence (verbal, physical and sexual) increases in probability. Sexual assaults often involve intoxicated perpetrators and victims. Socially these impacts are now well known and have an aggregating effect beyond the individuals concerned. Socio-economic resources are drawn upon and increase the tax burden as the emergency services, social services and the criminal justice system are implicated.

With this wider context of alcohol use in mind, how is its ubiquity across the lifespan played out differentially in older people? Some obvious points can be made. First, to have reached old age people have survived the mortality risk from the drug from younger days. They were not killed by a drunk driver and they did not die of cirrhosis of the liver or cardiac pathology in middle age. That survival may reflect their temperance or moderation, but not necessarily. Most heavy drinkers (around 80%) survive into old age with their livers intact, indicating a genetic bias in susceptibility to liver disease. The risk of cardiac pathology is also survived by many into old age, but middle-aged heart disease is correlated with the dose consumed (Fernández-Solà 2015).

Second, the life-long personal use of alcohol to lift the mood temporarily or relax the consumer is ingrained by old age. As all old habits die hard, direct appeals from public health or medical advice for moderation of abstinence may be ineffective. Moreover, alcohol has an analgesic effect and so may dull the physical pain of chronic or terminal conditions alone, or by potentiating the impact of prescribed or purchased drugs.

Third, older people have both the time and inclination to indulge themselves. During the day, when duties would have pre-empted the habit in younger days, they are free to do as they wish, provided they can access supplies of alcohol. Moreover, with old age comes the perennial consideration of the end of life, and so casual indulgences of consumption, from sweets and butter to alcohol and tobacco, may reflect a laissez-faire existential stance. This is the opposite side of the same coin of the very concerns that the medical profession has about risks to health in old age.

Older drivers might crash their cars more often and, in the home, alcohol affects balance and the risk of falls. With the concurrent risk of osteoporosis, especially in women, alcohol use is implicated in fractures, with the hip being the commonest. Alcohol use can also add to complications from pre-existing health conditions such as cardiac pathology, hypertension, strokes, vascular dementia and diabetes. This amplification of morbidities can be complicated further by the interactive effect of alcohol on prescribed medication. In older people taking several drugs ('polypharmacy') adding alcohol to the mix can have adverse experiential and behavioural impacts, many of which are unclearly determined and understood and will vary from one person to another.

With these basic points in mind, Box 8.1 provides a summary of public health concerns about problem drinking in older people.

Box 8.1 Problem drinking in older people

The public health concern has focused mainly on older people drinking in their own homes because of the increased physical risks it entails. Their presence in public drinking spaces is relatively rare because of mobility and sensory impairments (and maybe financial cost, given the relative poverty of many older people now out of the labour market). This raises the matter of relative social isolation, which in turn increases the probability of depressive symptoms. A biopsychosocial spiral then might emerge, as social withdrawal impacts psychological functioning, which in turn raises the probability of alcohol consumption.

For example, with the increasing prevalence of long-term health conditions aggregating with age, then alcohol can be a solace because of its analgesic and anxiolytic properties. Older adults suffering from multiple chronic morbidities and depression are nearly five times as likely to be problem drinkers as older adults with the same conditions and no depression. Such a correlational finding makes causality difficult to discern case by case. Do people (of any age) drink because they are depressed or does drinking lower mood between periods of inebriation? The causal relationship may not be linear but circular. The toxic effects of alcohol are debilitating and they lower mood. The existential state of recurring hangovers also might lower a person's sense of self-worth or exacerbate their sense of shame. That psychological pain is then relieved by more drinking and the vicious circle continues.

Another example of interactive causality relates to binge drinking, which increases by around a third in those retired. Social isolation may prompt a motivation to have a 'good time' when opportunities do arise to socialise with friends and family, such as holidays or family events.

Another example is about the loss of an intimate partner and peers from death. Mourning, especially when it is aggregating with years of individual survival may prompt an increase in alcohol consumption. The lower mood accruing can become entrenched and drinking is turned to, in order to numb the distress of isolation and loss on a daily basis. Aggregate mourning may also amplify social isolation because trusted social networks shrink and networks predict depression; thus becoming very old carries this double risk, with lone drinking being one option for comfort.

Experienced inequalities at the end of life

As we noted in Chapter 1, Therborn (2013) makes a distinction between *vital inequalities* (in relation to income, clean water, sanitation, shelter and a steady food supply) and *existential inequalities* (of respect and recognition). As people get older in all societies both or either of these can be under threat, within a national jurisdiction or region from person to person. Older people leave the labour market, with uneven retirement incomes and their recognition from others will be variable. If an increasing risk of physical and mental impairments is added to the picture, then existential inequalities tend to proliferate in old age. This is the context of differentiation in which we need to place Erickson's generic point about ego integrity versus despair. The tension the latter implies is partly an existential matter for individuals but their agency might be, to a range of degrees, impaired by cognitive decline and shaped by immediate social contingencies.

The subjective experience of death (not just its various causes) is also unevenly spread. For example, end-of-life care is inflected by affordability. The poor will not only die younger but their access to optimal palliative care be absent or limited if no state provision is available. In comparison the rich can buy optimal care, in terms of both residential facilities and paid carers.

For Erikson's generic point about the last phase of life being one of the tensions between ego integrity and despair, then the range of biological, psychological and social aspects of a particular individual arise relevant to consider. Biologically some emergent states may dominate that reflection (e.g., being diagnosed with a painful or debilitating terminal illness, loss of sight or hearing) or even alter the person's cognitive capacity to reflect at all. For those in the late stages of dementia that capacity may seem to disappear (at least to onlookers). The challenge then becomes the degree to which those around the demented patient are able and willing to afford them recognition.

If they do, is this giving due respect to a historical version of personhood, i.e., remembering the way the old person used to be and a recognition of their pre-dementing achievements?

Psychologically, despair may be warded off by the contingencies of remaining resources. These include the financial resources to enjoy life, the personal contacts retained to sustain well-being and the reckoning made internally about past achievements. Religion may be relevant as a source of succour in old age (with large personal variations in its salience for individuals).

Older people may be happy with their personal appraisal, or dissatisfied for a range of reasons. Collectively these might be 'existential guilt', which includes, a lack of fulfilled aspirations and feelings of guilt about what opportunities were missed or decisions made that are now regretted, as well as shame if, say, a good career was marred by a poor ending. Those not prone to feeling guilt or shame may defend against any negative emotional impact of their self-assessment.

The extent to which a person's social context affects their degree of despair in life will rely on both objective and subjective factors. Poverty (both relative and absolute) and threats from warfare impinge on old and young alike and so will be part of the picture of Erickson's phase described. Subjectively, people vary in their acceptance of these constrictions on life (religious belief noted might be a consideration here), alongside the impact of any additional burden of pain and impairment from disease, chronic or terminal, which increases in probability with age. One option if extreme despair is experienced, for all or any of the above reasons, is to commit suicide.

Although self-murder seems like a sudden break in our instinctive wish to survive, it might be seen to be on a continuum, throughout life but especially near to its end. The deliberate act of ending one's life occurs unevenly. Men (young as well as old) commit suicide more often than women. Given that the poor die younger and political instability or warfare inflect death rates, at any age, there are clear structural determinants at play. Elderly white men over the age of 85 years have the highest suicide rates (Conjero et al. 2016).

Risk factors for suicide include the presence of chronic pain and dependency on others, loneliness, feelings of abandonment and loss of meaning in life (Wand et al. 2019). In one recent qualitative study conditions that led older people to think about reasons behind suicide intent included social and cultural changes in society, a lack of social support, conflict in religious belief, the influence of economic uncertainty and socio-economic status, and depression as a result of the changes in people's social and domestic environments (Lydon et al. 2021).

Early death also emerges, in part, from self-injurious habits, such as excessive eating and tobacco and alcohol use and they in turn are class related. An example of political and economic shocks impacting on early mortality was the brutal shift in post-Soviet society from state socialism to neoliberalism, which led to the life expectancy of men dropping to 59 years of age. Many men literally 'drank themselves to death' with vodka. This continued a trend prior to the collapse of the USSR, with low birth rates and mass violent deaths, at the hands of both Hitler and Stalin (Brainerd 2021).

Finally, terminal illnesses such as untreatable cancer, heart failure or degenerative neurological conditions can affect people of any age, but they are commoner in older people. Consequently, the ethical and political contention about assisted dying and the right to commit suicide, in order to control one's biological end-point becomes more pertinent with age. Even without the presence of suffering from the impact of acute illness or degenerative conditions, requests for euthanasia or physician-assisted suicide are evident. One study showed a significant minority of people, who make such requests, do so on the basis primarily of being tired of living ('feeling bad', 'tired' and 'not active') (Rurup et al. 2005).

Conclusion

Our uneven chances of experiencing optimal physical and mental health are shaped by where we are in the life span. Matters of autonomy during early life are particularly important as the child or young person struggles to individuate in the face of psychosocial expectations. After retirement, there is the challenge of retaining a sense of well-being in the face of physical deterioration and loss of status. For some this is accompanied by loss of remuneration, meaning that poverty in old age is a particular threat to health and well-being.

If individuation is the existential challenge for the young, integration and reflections about biographical relevance face the old. The intersection of age and sex is particularly important to consider. Girls struggle more than boys with their mental health but men die younger than women and are more at risk of suicide. As with other variables we consider in this book, age as a source of inequality is important but not all important.

References

Abera, M., A. Nega, Y. Tefera, and A.A. Gelagay. 2020. "Early Marriage and Women's Empowerment: The Case of Child-Brides in Amhara National Regional State, Ethiopia." *BMC International Health & Human Rights* 20 (1): 30.

Ai-Bin, S.L. 2022. "From Developing to Developed: Mechanisms of Health Inequalities among Seniors in China and Japan under Macro-field Control." *Frontiers in Psychology* 5 (13): 956165.

Bernardi, F., M. Cozzani, and F. Zanasi. 2021. "Social Inequality and the Risk of Living in a Nursing Home: Implications for the COVID-19 Pandemic." *Genus* 77 (1): 9.

Blowers, L.C., et al. 2003. "The Relationship between Sociocultural Pressure to Be Thin and Body Dissatisfaction in Preadolescent Girls." *Eating Disorders* 4 (3): 229–224.

Brainerd, E. 2021. "Mortality in Russia since the Fall of the Soviet Union." *Comparative Economic Studies* 63: 557–576.

Brunskell-Evans, H., and M. Moore, eds. 2018. *Transgender Children and Young People: Born in Your Own Body*. Newcastle: Cambridge Scholars Publishing.

Cohen, D., and H. Barnes. 2019. "Gender Dysphoria in Children: Puberty Blockers Study Draws Further Criticism." *BMJ* 366: l5647.

Cohen, S. 1972. *Folk Devils and Moral Panics: The Creation of Mods and Rockers*. London: MacGibbon and Kee.

Conejero, I., J. Lopez-Castroman, L. Giner, and E. Baca-Garcia. 2016. "Sociodemographic Antecedent Validators of Suicidal Behavior: A Review of Recent Literature." *Current Psychiatry Reports* 18 (10): 94.

Drewnowski, A., C.L. Kurth, and D.D. Krahn. 1995. "Effects of Body Image on Dieting, Exercise, and Anabolic Steroid Use in Adolescent Males." *International Journal of Eating Disorders* 17 (4): 381–386.

Elks, M.L. 1994. "On the Genesis of Anorexia Nervosa – A Feminist Perspective." *Medical Hypothesis* 42: 180–182.

Emslie, C., and K. Hunt 2012. "Lyons a. older and Wiser? Men's and Women's Accounts of Drinking in Early Mid-life." *Sociology of Health & Illness* 34 (4): 481–496.

Fernández-Solà, J. 2015. "Cardiovascular Risks and Benefits of Moderate and Heavy Alcohol Consumption." *Nature Reviews. Cardiology* 12: 576–587.

Gilleard, C., and P. Higgs. 2009. "The Third Age: Field, Habitus or Identity?." In *Consumption and Generational Change: The Rise of Consumer Lifestyles and the Transformation of Later Life*, edited by I.R. Jones, P. Higgs, and D. Ekerdt, 61–75. New York: Transactions Press.

Higgs, G., M. Langford, and M. Llewellyn. 2022. "Towards an Understanding of Inequalities in Accessing Residential and Nursing Home Provision: The Role of Geographical Approaches." *Health & Social Care in the Community* 30 (6): 2218–2229.

Hoek, H.W., and D. van Hoeken. 2003. "Review of the Prevalence and Incidence of Eating Disorders." *International Journal of Eating Disorders* 34 (4): 383–396.

Kim, S., S.L. Spilman, D.H. Liao, P. Sacco, and A.A. Moore. 2018 Apr. "Social Networks and Alcohol Use Among Older Adults: A Comparison with Middle-aged Adults." *Aging Ment Health* 22 (4): 550–557. doi: 10.1080/13607863.2016.1268095. Epub 2016 Dec 22. PMID: 28006983; PMCID: PMC5523450.

Lloyd, S., J. Yiend, U. Schmidt, and K. Tchanturia. 2014. "Perfectionism in Anorexia Nervosa: Novel Performance Based Evidence." *PLOS ONE* 9 (10).

Lyndon, N., H. Azman, R.A. Che Rose, and M.F. Mat Jali. 2021. "Sociological Narratives of Suicidal Behavior among Older People." *Clinical Aging* 15(16): 1379–1392.

Solmi, F., S.L. Hatch, M. Hotopf, et al. 2014. "Prevalence and Correlates of Disordered Eating in a General Population Sample: The South East London Community Health (SELCoH) Study." *Social Psychiatry & Psychiatric Epidemiology* 49: 1335–1346.

Spilman, S.L., D.H. Liao, P. Sacco, and A.A. Moore. 2018. "Social Networks and Alcohol Use among Older Adults: A Comparison with Middle-Aged Adults." *Aging & Mental Health* 22 (4): 550–557.

Smink, F.R., D. van Hoeken, and H.W. Hoek. 2012. "Epidemiology of Eating Disorders: Incidence, Prevalence and Mortality Rates." *Current Psychiatry Reports* 14 (4): 406–414.

Therborn, G. 2013. *The Killing Fields of Inequality*. London: Polity Press.

Marcotte, D., L. Fortin, P. Potvin, and M. Papillon. 2002. "Gender Differences in Depressive Symptoms during Adolescents: Role of Gender-Typed Characteristics, Self-Esteem, Body Image, Stressful Life Evens, and Pubertal Status." *Journal of Emotional & Behavioral Disorders* 10 (1): 29–42.

MacGuire, F.A.S. 2020. "Reducing Health Inequalities in Aging through Policy Frameworks and Interventions." *Frontiers in Public Health* 8: 315. doi: 10.3389/fpubh.2020.00315. PMID: 32850574. PMCID: PMC7411218.

Orbach, S. 1986. *Hunger Strike: The Anorexic's Struggle as a Metaphor for Our Age*. London: Faber and Faber.

Parker, R., and S. Mauger. 1976. "Anorexia Nervosa." *Spare Rib* 28: 6–10.

Rogers, A., and D. Pilgrim. 2020. *A Sociology of Mental Health and Illness*, 6th edn. Buckingham: Open University Press.

Rurup, M.L., B.D. Onwuteaka-Philipsen, M.C. Jansen-van der Weide, and G. van der Wal. 2005. "When Being 'Tired of Living' Plays an Important Role in a Request for Euthanasia or Physician-Assisted Suicide: Patient Characteristics and the Physician's Decision." *Health Policy* 74 (2): 157–166. doi: 10.1016/j.healthpol.2005.01.002.

Samaras, T.T., L.H. Storms, and H. Elrick. 2002. "Longevity, Mortality and Body Weight." *Ageing Research Reviews* 1 (4): 673–691.

Vander Wal, J.S., and M.H. Thelen. 2000. "Predictors of Body Image Dissatisfaction in Elementary-Age School Girls." *Eating Behaviors* 1 (2): 105–122.

Volpe, U., A. Tortorella, M. Manchia, A.M. Monteleone, U. Albert, and P. Monteleone. 2016. "Eating Disorders: What Age at Onset?." *Psychiatry Research* 238: 225–227.

Wand, A.P.F., B. Draper, H. Brodaty, and C. Peisah. 2019. "Self-Harm in the Very Old One Year Later: Has Anything Changed?." *International Journal of Geriatric Psychiatry* 31: 1559–1568.

Wiles, J.L., A. Leibing, N.Guberman, J. Reeve, and R.E. Allen. 2021. "The Meaning of 'Aging in Place' to Older People." *Gerontologist* 52 (3): 357–366.

Wysokiński, A., T. Sobów, I. Kłoszewska, and T. Kostka. 2015. "Mechanisms of the Anorexia of Aging-A Review." *Age (Dordrecht, Netherlands)* 37 (4): 9821.

Young, J. 1971. *The Drugtakers: The Social Meaning of Drug Use*. London: Judson. McGibbon and Kee.

9 Pandemics
The great un-levelling?

Introduction

Recently the spread of Coronavirus disease, Covid-19, has dominated our awareness as a shared challenge. This final chapter considers that seemingly universal 'all in the same boat' character. Much has been written about this most recent pandemic, some but by no means all of which is mentioned below. However, our intention is not to offer an immediate and comprehensive review of commentary and research, but instead highlight themes that have been common throughout this book, in relation to living with inequalities. The extent and quality of the first-response attempt to research the infection are yet to be appraised.

Some of the emergent themes now accumulating in the literature, relate to infectious diseases, preceded the Covid-19 pandemic and were then illuminated further by its recent emergence. For example, the emergence of AIDS in the 1980s was an important similar occurrence and, before that, the 'Spanish flu' of 1918 occurred. Pandemics create grave immediate threat to life and many create chronic ongoing disability (we consider 'long Covid' below in the context of more mundane and less considered forms of post-viral conditions).

The impacts of morbidity and mortality under conditions of pandemic are accompanied by abrupt and dramatic implications for the economy, the development of science and wider society. Beyond the direct pressure on healthcare for acute cases, the imposed lockdown of Covid-19 altered daily relationality for all people (with some members of the elite being accused at times of arrogant exceptionalism in their personal conduct).

The spectre of a potentially collapsing economy was accompanied by draconian measures of increased State control. In some countries the police and the military enforced lockdowns, with ordinary people protesting, when these measures seemed nonsensical or disproportionate. The most vulnerable in society became even more vulnerable. These included those with no fixed abode and the precarious, such as migrant workers, the inmates of prisons, care and retail staff, transport workers and the entrapped victims of abuse in domestic settings. The practical *opportunity* to stay at home and stay safe, or keep a safe distance in public, was not on offer in an equal way in daily

DOI: 10.4324/9781003025641-9

life. In the wider context of uneven forms of exposure to infection, financial markets became volatile, and mass unemployment was threatened.

Thus pandemics can then be framed as complex biopsychosocial 'critical situations' and are a prism through which to observe the playing out of pre-existing inequalities in everyday life. State-sponsored and public-health measures designed to mitigate viral spread, and its consequences, created social divisions that impacted not only on peoples' physical health, but also their emotional and social well-being. However, this impact was not uniform in fashion. Below we consider three particular aspects of the recent pandemic: the ways in which it amplified and drew attention to pre-existing inequalities; the ambivalence of some in the population about vaccine policy compliance, the position and views of those who are marginalised within this and the matter of trust in authority; and the unequal consideration of post-viral fatigue, when Covid-19 is compared to other infections.

An empirical summary of Covid-19 and tentative lessons learned

The personal and interpersonal effects of Covid-19 threw a spotlight on why the psychosocial aspects of the disease are as salient to understand as its biological character and containment. Covid-19 has not only been about whether or not health anxiety rises or falls from person to person during a pandemic. The disease also disrupted interpersonal routines and peoples' views of others through moralisations about compliance and non-compliance to protect others, not just the self. 'Risky' conduct, which became linked in public health advice to becoming infected, led at times to 'victim blaming', when choices were constrained for some of us more than others. Ordinary negative psychosocial processes, such as panic contagion and stigma, came into play but also a background fear of death became foregrounded (Strong 1990).

This anxiety-laden situation prompted the use of war metaphors, which in turn reinforced the need for compliance with a-typical measures of mass social control over everyday lives. Covid-19 was not new in this regard. In the case of AIDS there were moralisations about sexual promiscuity, which took root in language-pervading prevention strategies for gay and bisexual men, even though social-cognitive approaches stressing individual responsibility for health proved to be largely ineffective (Halkitis 2019). A foreboding British government advertising campaign in 1986 warned us all not to 'die of ignorance'. This triggered secondary controversies about homophobia, when a 'gay plague' was the common discourse in the mass media.

More recently in relation to Covid-19, health promotion language emphasised action against the threat as requiring a *collective* endeavour in war against the disease (e.g., isolation). However, the capacity to comply equally was missing. As we have already noted above, the sociopsychological impact of newly justified and introduced policies varied from one social group to another.

Pandemics exacerbate differences in living circumstances, restricting already restricted lives even further. Taken-for-granted sources of joy or the vitality found in everyday conviviality in public spaces were severely curtailed. Restrictions brought in as a result of the pandemic were inevitably the product of attempts to prevent the spread of the virus by the state, via public health measures of distancing and isolation. These controls and policy arrangements intensified pre-existing challenges of navigating the institutional settings of school, workplaces and the built environment in particular ways. An example here was the distress surrounding restricted visiting arrangements of those in hospitals or care facilities. In other words, people were discovering not only the challenges about personal hygiene and risk avoidance or minimisation, they also ran up against the constraints of institutions and their particular rules. Public spaces took on a new salience (e.g., about entering shops or shared buildings or getting on a bus) in ways not previously noticeable. Taken-for-granted access and mobility in these spaces suddenly became a source of anxious consideration, testing our concentration and confidence.

Pandemics and the amplification of inequalities

The nineteenth-century physician William Farr noted the way in which disease epidemics:

> infest the habitations of the poor, and strike the artisan in his strength down from comfort into helpless poverty; they carry away the infant from the mother's breast, and the old man at the end of life.
>
> (William Farr 1856, 76 cited in Armstrong 2021)

Farr considered that inequalities in mortality were seen as originating from 'natural deaths', now accelerated by want and privations, such as what he noted in particular were 'intemperance and starvation'. Likewise we can see that the recent Covid-19 pandemic replicated, amplified and accelerated existing inequalities in mortality and morbidity. Obesity, economic deprivation, poor living conditions and ethnicity are all relevant factors in to consider in this regard.

People in low-income communities were more likely to have become unwell. In many countries Black and ethnic minority communities experienced significantly higher risk of serious illness or death from the virus. So too with older people in care homes and families in restricted domestic situations. Caring for children in low-income neighbourhoods, with high population density was high risk for adults, with the latter being more at risk the older they were.

Covid-19 was, in part, a respiratory disease at least in its symptom profile. Accordingly, those already affected by environmental pollution in and around the home, which we discussed in Chapter 4, were placed at increased risk (Bray et al. 2020). Those living in neighbourhoods of increased deprivation, already in contact with welfare services were prone to additional challenges (Patrick et al. 2022). Thus, viewed through the lens of the ecology of risk, we see that place was an important aspect of understanding the impact of Covid-19. But it also implicated demographic factors within localities. The multi-factorial social patterning of risk is summarised in Box 9.1.

Box 9.1 The social patterning of the pandemic

- *Place*: Covid-19 prevalence was higher in those living in more deprived circumstances.
- *Existing morbidity*: Those with underlying health conditions such as diabetes, COPD or cardiovascular problems were at higher risk of death or severe acute symptoms. Women were more likely to be diagnosed with Covid-19 than men. Men were more likely to die from the acute infection.
- *Ethnicity*: The highest rates of diagnosis of Covid-19 were in Black and ethnic minority groups. The lowest were in people of White ethnic groups. Those of Bangladeshi ethnicity had twice the risk of death compared to people of White British ethnicity. People of Chinese, Indian, Pakistani, Other Asian, Caribbean and Other Black ethnicity had between 10% and 50% higher risk of death when compared to White British (Dey and Sinha 2020).
- *Occupational status*: For those already at home (outside of the labour market) isolation pre-existed. For those in some white-collar jobs, working from home became a new norm. Some other groups such as care workers and those in retail work or public transport, were at high risk of infection.
- *Long Covid* sufferers report a set of fluctuating symptoms, including fatigue, breathlessness, chest pain, post-exercise malaise, cognitive dysfunction. Long Covid impacts those of older age, high body mass index (BMI), smoking, being female, those living in the most socio-economically deprived areas and those with public-facing jobs (Razieh et al. 2023).

Multi-factorial intersectionality explanatory focus

The content of Box 9.1 summarises examples of the social patterning of Covid-19. It is useful to see aspects of the differences that are illuminated, as part of the impact of the pandemic. Each discrete variance could be accounted for separately; in relation to sex, by women having more exposure during Covid-19 in the caring and retail roles than men but seemingly lower rates of mortality. Women tend to die less than men from acute viral infections (Mauvais-Jarvis et al. 2020; Moelem 2020). Reductionist explanations about particular social group membership are limited and causal interactions seem to be understood better in some social contexts than others and it has been suggested that explanations of a multi-factorial picture are probably best seen through the lens of intersectionality (Bowleg 2020). This way of looking at things reveals more about how interlocking aspects of power and inequality are structured for groups of people who prior to Covid-19 have a legacy of being oppressed, predicated on an interwoven set of demographics (race, ethnicity, sex, class). The racial and ethnic differences are complicated by poverty and locale (Wacquant 2022). The unequal impact on communities includes social and economic inequalities, poor housing, entrenched structural and institutional racism, discrimination stigma, higher occupational risk exposure, the prevalence of conditions increasing the severity of disease – obesity, diabetes, cardiovascular disease (CVD) and asthma, and poorer access to and experiences of health care and individual and community exposure to Covid-19 (Nazroo and Becares 2020).

When considering the complex of influences it is likely that locality, sex, age, class and ethnicity and pre-existing poverty of resourceful networks have a multiplying effect when disadvantaged situations intersect (Kovacs et al. 2021). This pattern of access to health and social-care support was replicated across different countries during the pandemic. Those already frail, sick or disabled were made worse in a negative spiral of physical pain, psychological distress, lack of financial resources and social isolation (Fallon et al. 2021). In some isolated rural villages in Italy, during lockdown, older people were reported not only to be dying of the virus but also of starvation (Rudin 2020).

The funding and differential access to healthcare added to the complexity. For example, in California Latino patients with Covid-19, and those on Medicaid, were more likely to present to emergency care and to enter inpatient settings, compared to those with private insurance. The latter were more likely to be dealt with successfully in an outpatient location, whereas those poorer patients presenting to emergency care were more likely to die from the infection (Vaughn et al. 2021). It is ambiguous whether these differences in mortality rate reflected the extant vulnerability of poorer patients or the differential clinical risks of the two settings or whether these combined in some way. The intersection of multiple factors might also be relevant to the long-term impacts of Covid-19. These are inflected by age, body mass index, sex, smoking status, poverty and occupation (Shabnam et al. 2022).

Living daily life and social position

The occupational dimension to the effects of Covid-19 was compounded by the differences in the living arrangements which were partially determined by the jobs that people do. During the pandemic exposure to risk and clinical outcomes divided starkly along the lines of socio-material status. Lowly paid workers were dramatically exposed and included those in health and social-caring occupations, particularly nursing and care-home staff. Added risks accrued to those transporting passengers, such as bus drivers and taxi or minicab drivers. So too with those working in retail frontline and security guards (Rozenfeld et al. 2020).

Middle-class people were more likely to have access to gardens and personal outdoor space. Their shopping options were also more flexible. Disadvantaged poorer families were more likely to be furloughed with fewer luxuries and less wealth to rely on to buy essentials. Some were forced into queues for access to supermarkets but there was home delivery from upmarket supermarkets for others.

This recreated the circumstances of the late nineteenth century, when shopping was often delivered to the better-off by a 'delivery' boy in a horse and cart or on a bicycle. Moreover, home deliveries of those protected at home were brought by lower-paid workers who were then in a position of being more exposed to the virus through multiple contacts. The customer was exposed once in such an interaction but the worker delivering the groceries was exposed to every customer each working day and another group the next.

The extent to which the practicalities and comforts of home working enhanced working, leisure and domestic life was shaped by the space of home and garden. In the UK, the virus prompted a shift to more desirable living arrangements for those who could afford it (https://www.theguardian.com/world/2020/sep/26/escape-country-covid-exodus-britain-cities-pandemic-urban-green-space). The interest that the mass media took in the pandemic also shaped as well as responded to public perceptions. Journalists relayed research and surveys in their reporting.

For example, one such report was of the UK Covid Social Study, which asked 70,000 people what they thought of lockdown. This study pointed out 'dramatic changes' in people's lives (particularly in relation to loneliness and mental health: https://www.covidsocialstudy.org). News reports in the pandemic, unlike the press reporting characterised by victim blaming of those leading unhealthy lives that we discussed in the early chapters of the book, sympathetically highlighted the emergence of inequalities and the reasons why these occurred. For example, a seemingly unlikely source of this sociological comparison, and value judgements about it, was from *Newsnight* on BBC2 television, from which we cite here its lead presenter Emily Maitlis (20 April 2020):

> They tell us the coronavirus is a great leveller ... it's much harder if you are poor. The language around Covid has sometimes felt trite and misleading. You do not survive the virus through fortitude and strength of character, whatever the prime minister's colleagues tell us ... And the disease is not a great leveller the consequences of which rich and poor suffer the same. This is a myth which needs debunking ... Those on the

> front line right now bus drivers, shelf stackers, nurses, care home workers, shop keepers are disproportionately the lower paid of our workforce. They are more likely to catch the disease because they are more exposed. Those in tower blocks and small flats will find the lockdown a lot tougher. Those who work in manual jobs will be unable to work from home. The health issue has huge ramifications for social welfare and it's a huge social issue with ramifications for public health. We ask what sort of settlement needs to be put in place to stop inequalities becoming even more stark.

The usually conservative *Daily Telegraph* newspaper also commented negatively and somewhat moralistically on the disparity trend:

> It feels like a dirty secret – that middle-class lives should have actually improved, even as others less fortunate have disproportionately lost their jobs, relationships and lives.

It goes on:

> While furloughed workers in the hospitality sector, say – used to getting all the exercise they needed on their feet all day at work – piled on the pounds on the couch at home; flush work-from-homers were able to splash out on digital exercise apps, gadgets and services.
>
> (https://www.telegraph.co.uk/family/life/meet-covid-comfortables-middle-classes-got-richer-pandemic/)

This link with exercise was also echoed by findings from a survey by the Institute for Social and Economic Research, which found a correlation with income. Those on lower incomes reported exercising less, as a result of having less space, inside and out as a means to get fit (Eliott et al. 2022). The *Financial Times* reported on the privileged health gains of bankers able to spend more time practicing for marathons and exercising in home gyms with the assistance of high-tech bicycles and fitness apps.

> One banker interviewed stated: 'It's definitely [due to] having more time,' he says, describing his midweek exercise as 'hit and miss' in the pre-Covid-19 world of commuting, frequent business trips and meeting-packed schedules.
>
> (https://www.ft.com/content/2d7dc42d-4c88-4e17-89d3-9bf604fe88b1)

The unusual concerns of sections of the media with social class appear to be a novelty thrown up by the pandemic. One possibility is that the middle-class workforce was enjoying 'too much' autonomy in the wake of the new situation, reflecting a concern about productivity from commentators about a loss of routine workplace discipline, under the traditional direct surveillance of managers. (This question of the productivity of home versus office working is one of many uncertainties left by post-pandemic in the context of only a partial return to routine working outside of the home.)

This picture of hyper-exposure compared unfavourably, in terms of risk of infection, with workers with less exposure (see below), greater wealth and quality of life. Overall, middle- to higher-income households acquired *savings* through the pandemic and their homeworking ensured their greater safety and living a better life. Their salaries were maintained but their commuting costs were temporarily eliminated. In contrast, those on low wages had no savings' pot to protect against any new costs incurred or loss of earnings because of redundancy, as well as being more likely to be in occupational groups with a raised risk of infection (/www.resolutionfoundation.org/app/uploads/2021/01/Pandemic-pressures.pdf think tank).

State-sponsored measures also fed into the occupational constellation of fortune for the middle classes. Lockdown as a policy entailed the closure of small businesses, local services and schools, causing economic hardship and stress for everyone to some extent, but for some much more than for others. As we have just noted, for the middle classes, in line with a history of more autonomous work roles, it permitted greater freedom to work from home. Whether one was able to work from home or not depended on the occupation and norms of the advantages conferred by professional autonomy. The degree of the latter was reported in pre-pandemic times as a relevant factor in the development of illness: a lack of control over work content tasks leads to increased stress and this has psychosomatic consequences. For example, Marmot and colleagues (1997) demonstrated in their research how most of the inverse social gradient in the incidence of heart disease amongst different grades of civil servants could be attributed to differences in psychosocial work environments in relation to task control. This trend of the pre-pandemic driver of the risk of illness was amplified by the biopsychosocial complexity of Covid-19. We now move on to a particular focus thrown into relief by the pandemic: variable vaccine uptake and vaccine hesitancy.

Vaccine hesitancy and the politics of trust revealed in a pandemic

'Being afraid' is a core aspect of pandemics. This creates a bind for the frightened. What if an offer of prevention itself creates fear? This is called an 'avoidance–avoidance conflict', i.e., whatever option we choose, there may be dire consequences, which we wish to avoid (Lewin 1935). The mass availability of vaccines, rapidly produced and for many relieved mass anxiety created by a virus spreading death and illness. However, whilst it relieved anxiety for many it invoked one anxiety amongst many others, which stemmed from the deliberate introduction of a pharmaceutical substance into, what for now, was an uninfected body.

This non-compliance with vaccination when offered is a long-standing focus in public health discussions and has often been a contested matter in relation to childhood vaccination programmes where babies and children are not able to provide consent (or withhold it) (Rogers and Pilgrim 1995). During Covid-19 children were the least at risk and were not the initial targets of the vaccination programme, and adults had full capacity to agree with the intervention. For the rationalists, confident in the low risks involved, this was a 'no brainer' and rates of uptake were high. As many people as possible should be and were vaccinated when offered, as soon as possible, in order to protect themselves and others. Mass vaccination was generally free for any groups identified and so resistance was not about financial cost to the individual recipient. Some older people were anxious to get another dose as soon as possible to reduce their health anxiety. Despite this rationale for free protection from the infection, doubts for some were introduced on a number of fronts and whilst on the face of things vaccine hesitancy – delay in acceptance or refusal of vaccination despite its availability – appeared to be a binary decision of acceptance or refusal the issue itself, it's expression and consequences were socially patterned. In Britain the expression of the likelihood of taking up the offer of a vaccine was lower amongst young people, those with fewer years of education, women, members of lower-income households and of other than White ethnic groups (Callaghan et al. 2021)

What actually happened in practice was, of course, complex. Compliance varied from person to person and by social group membership. Some nations were far more compliant than others. Conspiracy theories emerged, but what if there were real economic and political interests at play, which might actually imply that conspiracies, or at least manipulation, by elites and the government were genuinely present? After all, if they were then the last thing that the elite beneficiaries would do is to admit what was going on. Whether these perceived negative forces and risk to self from vaccination were warranted or merely lurid fantasies, or any stop in between, what matters is that beliefs about nefarious interest work took on a social reality for some and became motives for personal resistance and action.

The 'pro' versus 'anti' positions touched on and illuminated several areas about trust or distrust of the drug companies, health professionals and governments. Those in favour of compliance showed a willingness to accept the integrity and wisdom of this trio, whereas 'anti-vaxxers' had the opposite viewpoint. However, ambivalence was also present. For example, some people were cynical about drug company profiteering but also very keen to minimise risk to self, because the public health advice was trusted in principle. In the case of the UK, traditional trust in the NHS ensured high compliance rates. Indeed, some complaints emerged about local variations in the availability of the vaccine. However, for some groups (e.g., other than White ethnic groups) the opposite effect was evident. Some did not want the vaccine because they had a pre-existing lack of trust in government, scientists and health professionals (Allington et al. 2022).

The motives for suspicion were varied and aggregated in individual cases. In the other direction, those keen to promote mass vaccination pointed to anti-science elements in society, who were keen to undermine traditional governmental authority, pumping misinformation into social media (see e.g., https://www.bma.org.uk/news-and-opinion/pushing-back-tackling-the-anti-vax-movement).

For the marginalised and disadvantaged, the matter of vaccine hesitancy, where it occurred, may have reflected a subjective f continuity, in relation to experienced power differentials, lack of control, stigma and discrimination, experienced *previously* in relation to healthcare systems and professionals. These aspects have been well documented as aspects of unequal access to or negative experiences with services (Rogers and Pilgrim 2003) and resonate with personal ambivalence about compliance with authority at the time of Covid-19.

Thus, vaccine hesitancy may be influenced by a relationship to institutional authority. Middle- and working-class mothers seem to feel personal power and constraints differently in choosing to be vaccinated or not, which has an influence on what actions they think they can take. This is evident in a study in which working-class mothers expressed fears that health and educational professionals might act as reporters for state intervention (e.g., Child Protection Services) and experienced push back by health professionals as coercion.

> I felt very scare-tactic'd into [vaccines]. Without so many words, 'You're going to kill your children. You're a bad mom and you need to do this. I'm a doctor, I know better.'
>
> (Rogers and Pilgrim 1995)

By contrast, middle-class mothers did not express such concerns and felt less uncomfortable in refusing vaccines in spite of an awareness of social judgements being made and the repetitious and insistent appeals to vaccinate they were exposed to. The pandemic vaccine refusal is likely to have been underpinned by an ability of middle-class parents to be confident and construct, promote and articulate elaborate rationales for refusing vaccines. The latter private resilience to vaccine uptake campaigns, by more self-confident service users, is in the context of the heated and forceful way in which non-compliance is treated more generally in public. For example, the mainstream media ran pieces vilifying those 'refusing' vaccines (Glassman and Szymczak 2022).

Vaccine hesitancy can be seen as being linked to the growing power imbalances that were part of people's lives lived during the time of the pandemic. A study undertaken in Bradford (UK) suggested that the greater the perplexity, distress and mistrust about the nature of social worlds prior to the pandemic the less positive people seemed to be about being offered vaccines (Lockyer et al. 2021). The matter of vaccine hesitancy was also salient for the most marginalised care workers and lowly paid healthcare workers – those working at the coal face with first-hand experience of the health crises of Covid-19 and how it was being managed. A lack of trust in authorities seemingly fuelled vaccine hesitancy. A qualitative study suggests scepticism about the way Covid-19 deaths were reported and mistrust over hospitalisation statistics (exaggerated compared with accounts from those working in clinical settings).

> There was little to no help from the government. I think we were completely and utterly failed in terms of PPE … now the government want to try and make us have it [the vaccine] that's made me feel really like I don't want to.
>
> (Dennis et al. 2022)

In some countries there were cultural reasons feeding into feeling disempowered, related to the past, which influenced decision-making. For example, in post-Communist Bulgaria, there remains a cynicism about government, amplified by a norm of corruption post-transition since the 1990s (Boytchev 2021). Despite its free availability vaccine uptake there was poor during the Covid-19 pandemic. Bulgaria had the lowest rate in Europe (only 28% uptake) and, to confirm the mainstream rationalist position, it also had the highest death rate from the disease. Cynicism about government corruption recently, and older resentments about top-down authoritarianism under Communism, have encouraged a strong norm of individual rights, especially the basic right just to say 'no' (https://bnr.bg/en/post/101552479).

Wariness in Bulgaria was amplified by other perceptions from ordinary people. Why was vaccination being offered for free, when other pharmaceutical products were unaffordable for the bulk of the population? This cultural and economic context in which vaccines were being viewed in Bulgaria might account for the paradox that something that was being given free by the state to protect the individual was being refused by the majority. These considerations in both Eastern and Western Europe pointed out class differences in those who were vaccine refusers. Richer refusers were contemptuous of those who criticised them (maybe even invoking pride in their stubborn position). By contrast, poor and more marginalised people were more likely to feel a mixture of fear that they are being manipulated and anger that it was happening at all.

Recovery from the effects of pandemics and managing in the longer term

When the acute phase is over, pandemics continue to have lasting physical, psychological and social impacts. Medical and social resources are required for coping with the long-term impact of living with the daily consequences of pandemics now dissipated. This has implications for the focus of this book on inequalities in a range of ways. Both the pandemics of HIV and Covid-19 illuminate the point and will be considered in turn. In previous chapters we have illuminated the vagaries of daily life in inequalities in terms of the experience of the risk of long-term conditions. The status of the suffering of those with chronic conditions out with pandemics is more prevalent amongst those who are marginalised and is relevant here in relation to the matter of long-term fatigue and other symptoms. The unequal presentation of the two similar conditions is a matter of knowledge production and deployment. The general public are subjected to these aspects of applied expert knowledge and they may then trust or distrust what is being asked of them.

Lessons from self-care patient education for HIV as a long-term condition

In the Western world men who have sex with men were more likely to suffer from AIDS than women. After the acute phase at the end of the 1990s this pattern became clear. Injecting drug users were also a group at higher risk. Men who have sex with men were estimated to acquire HIV at rates 44 times greater than other men and 40 times greater than women (CDC 2011, https://www.cdc.gov/hiv/library/factsheets/index.html). Multiple social and contextual factors persisted in living with HIV over time. Economic disadvantage, neighbourhood characteristics, housing instability, incarceration, transactional sex, multiple partners, substance abuse and age at first intercourse were identified as risk factors. Reducing socio-economic disadvantage, provision of housing stability and condom use were then identified as protective factors for HIV exposure (Silva et al. 2022).

Given the high mortality rate in the acute phase of the pandemic, therapeutic pessimism prevailed for a while. However, slowly treatment improvements were made and living with, rather than dying from, AIDS became commoner amongst those infected with HIV. Bio-medical interventions decreased viral load and this improved outcomes for many. The diagnosis was no longer a death sentence and it had become the challenge of living with chronic symptoms and stigma. Continuing to live with HIV played out differently for different groups.

At the height of the HIV pandemic, vulnerabilities driven by homophobia were exacerbated for gay men, who might be burdened by other social circumstances of racism and poverty and common discrimination based on sexuality (Agenor et al. 2019). Living with HIV, over the longer term, seemingly extends the personal impact of the accumulation of experiences of prejudice. In extreme cases, this can trigger a sense of hopelessness and the perception of having a HIV status as being a personal failure. This in turn may mean a withdrawal from social life and a retreat into loneliness (Ferlatti et al. 2022).

Living with being HIV positive over time has become a long-term condition requiring everyday management. Take the example of a study of this heterogeneous group in the North West of England (Kennedy et al. 2007). This was an ethnography of people who were HIV+ and were attending a course on managing their long-term condition. Group members came together from different backgrounds but had a shared connection of becoming infected during and after the 1980s. The mainly gay male attendees were part of an age cohort, which had pushed back hard against the homophobic stigma at the outset of the AIDS pandemic. They included activists advocating appropriate and acceptable responses from government and policy-makers.

By contrast, the other course members were recently arrived heterosexual female asylum-seekers, mainly from war zones in sub-Saharan Africa. They had lived with the threat and consequences of HIV in one environment for some time and in another for a much shorter period. The immediate social-existential concerns for these women were different from the men in the group. The former focused on the anxious legal challenges of successful asylum seeking. The latter were concerned with daily living challenges and personal and interpersonal adjustments about their long-term condition. The former talked of their recent instability in a part of the world, where they were poor and stigmatised, as well as being civilians in a war zone. They also discussed a lack of healthcare and their dealings with traditional healers. This wider distress was discussed, whereas the men reported in a more focused way about a trajectory of coping and de-stigmatisation since the diagnosis, as well as new challenges arising with the process of ageing.

The group then had members who were seemingly in the 'same boat', by dent of their common infection, but with quite different concerns about its implications. The focus of the course they were all attending was on self-efficacy when living with a long-term condition. The accounts from the two subgroups revealed different and even diverging social-existential challenges. For the women the latter were less about the disease itself and more about social acceptance and ontological insecurity in an ambivalent host society. The self-efficacy emphasis left unaddressed pressing social, administrative and material needs. Despite these differences, sharing the different experiences living with the chronic condition and the contexts of its origin, meant that there was an increased mutual empathy between the two subgroups recorded by the researchers. The changing trajectory of AIDS as a longer term condition resonates with the sequela of Covid-19.

The lessons of 'long Covid'

Those with 'long Covid' report a set of fluctuating symptoms, including fatigue, breathlessness, chest pain, post-exercise malaise and cognitive dysfunction or 'brain fog'. The quality of life of some suffering from long Covid has been equated to those with stage 4 lung cancer (Walker et al. 2023).

Ten to 30% of people who became symptomatic with Covid-19 are estimated to still be experiencing long-lasting debilitating symptoms from the infection. These include extreme tiredness and shortness of breath, greater levels of anxiety, depression, physical inactivity, social strain and a lack of availability of sources of positive social support. At times this phenomenon, as with other impacts of the pandemic, has been depicted as 'unprecedented'. For the National Institute of Health Research in the UK, 'long Covid' is presented as the 'next big global challenge' and is noted as a *new* disease requiring extensive new investment in research and management options (https://evidence.nihr.ac.uk/themedreview/researching-long-covid-addressing-a-new-global-health-challenge/).

Following the logic of this purportedly new challenge, research must be wide-ranging. Many urgent questions seemingly remain unanswered. Who is most at risk of developing the condition? What is its underlying biology? And which medical treatments and rehabilitation techniques will help patients return to their daily tasks and normal well-being? This marks out 'long Covid' by its exceptionalism. However, that assumption is questionable for a number of reasons, which have already been evidenced in the literature on chronic conditions, prior to the outbreak of the pandemic.

In particular depicting 'long Covid' as being a brand-new health policy challenge, risks ignoring a body of knowledge about experienced fatigue, pain and fluctuating symptoms associated with many long-term conditions, especially those triggered by a viral infection. As with these other conditions, those now suffering from 'long Covid' report varied symptoms, some of which are not disease-specific. Neat clinical categories are not necessarily helpful guides to either understanding chronic fatigue or promoting coping strategies for those affected. There are exceptions to this rule, but those with differing long-term conditions report overlapping daily living challenges.

For example, the research findings we have on those with a diagnosis of 'chronic fatigue syndrome' (CFS) or 'ME' (myalgic encephalomyelitis) suggest a similar profile to that of 'long Covid'. This involves 'unexplained' fatigue lasting for more than six months, headaches, unrefreshing sleep, muscle pain and memory and concentration problems (Bhui et al. 2011). The individuals reporting this mixture of debilitating symptoms then face a range of practical problems. These include a lack of motivation to deal with daily tasks, the inability to travel far from the house and potential stigma. The latter refers to anyone with vague symptoms affecting motivation and competence. For example, it might be accounted in the eyes of cynical others by laziness or the secondary gain of being in the sick role. Affected patients may be wary to disclose too much about their experiences for fear of this sort of stigmatisation.

Thus a new challenge of the management of self is posed for the person that was not present before they were infected. They are expected to have recovered and to be returning to their old roles and responsibilities, but this is difficult to achieve and this can trigger demoralisation or depression. The latter then amplifies the primary motivational challenge and so a negative spiral may be created. The person may feel a mixture of shame, confusion and anger about their state. This complex picture of subjective distress might also have direct occupational and so financial consequences. If a person cannot return to their work then they lose both money and social status (if the latter is valued by them and others). We see here then a mix of problems for those with any post-viral residual effects (Peters et al. 2009).

The implications of this post-viral picture vary from one social group to another and between those times which are labelled as a pandemic and other times, which are not. Those in middle-class high-status occupations may be particularly sensitive to loss of status and identity, even though it can affect anyone recovering from Covid-19 or many other viral infections. Their profile in media reporting may have been one reason that 'long Covid' has been reified as a new condition and is seen as being 'unprecedented', to use the cliché now associated with the recent pandemic.

This news report of a woman with long Covid illustrates the point:

> Susan, aged 63, is a health policy consultant who considered herself fit and healthy before catching COVID-19 in April 2020. At that time, she was an avid hill walker and regularly practised yoga.
>
> (https://www.who.int/europe/news/item/09-08-2022-a-life-altered-by-long-covid---susan-s-experience)

The portrayed exceptionalism of 'long Covid' is in some ways understandable in the context of so many sudden symptoms and people suffering with the onset of the pandemic. The experience was traumatic for those who were previously well and healthy.

> I loved my job, had good friends and felt as high as a kite on life. Then I got Covid-19, and nothing prepared me for what happened next. As the illness developed, I felt so unwell I thought I was dying. The roller-coaster that followed lasted for months, with sudden waves of illness and malaise, like being hit by a cricket bat. I had a foggy head, acutely painful calf, upset stomach, tinnitus, aching all over, breathlessness, dizziness, arthritis in my hands, weird sensation in my skin, extreme emotions, and utter exhaustion and body aches throughout. I had ringing in my ears, intermittent changes to my heartbeat, and dramatic mood swings. After three months I was unable to be out of bed for more than three hours at a stretch. My arms and legs were permanently fizzing. I wondered: was the virus still there? Or did I have ME/CFS?
>
> (https://blogs.bmj.com/bmj/2021/01/25/paul-garner-on-his-recovery-from-long-covid/)

However, its treatment as something exceptional was also brought into doubt by some early research, which has compared it with those with a diagnosis of CFS or ME (Jason et al. 2021). This indicated that the acute challenges of Covid-19 were more pronounced than other flu-like conditions, but that those with CFS or ME suffered hard to shift symptoms over more months and years. In comparison, the 'long Covid' group seemed to be showing less chronicity, with more evidence of gradual improvement. As the researchers reported: 'over time, the long-hauliers evidenced significantly less severe symptoms than those with ME/CFS, except in the orthostatic domain' (Jason et al. 2021). (The latter is a reference to persistent low blood pressure, which is often linked to experienced tiredness.)

If 'long Covid' is not unique then it might be beneficial to learn about its amelioration from previous research on other long-term conditions. The lessons learned from the latter can be applied quite reasonably. Depicting it as a new condition or 'unprecedented' may misdirect health policy and research. Wheels might be re-invented unnecessarily. Moreover, if that prior literature is a point of reference, then as the ethnographic report on the AIDS group noted earlier, maybe the differentiations to be made are not about the biology of infections but their variegates psycho-social implications.

This returns us to inequalities. Indeed, the media reports of 'long Covid' on the standing and capabilities of middle-class professionals (see earlier) will raise the salience of one affected group and ignore its presence in, and impact upon, the less well-off. Those who are poor and marginalised may be relatively ignored. This risk is already apparent in the literature addressing chronic conditions, other than 'long Covid', from previous knowledge about the impact of post-viral states.

For example, poorer people with a diagnosis of CFS have particular or amplified psychosocial challenges, which may not routinely be taken seriously by healthcare systems and professionals (Kingstone et al. 2020). To finish on a recurring point that includes the focus on long Covid – the suspicion is that those who are middle class or better-off have had a more privileged experience in pandemic conditions: 'Whisper it, but Britain's own middle class has done quite nicely out of Covid' (https://www.telegraph.co.uk/family/life/meet-covid-comfortables-middle-classes-got-richer-pandemic/).

Conclusion

We remain too close to the Covid-19 pandemic to draw strong conclusions about its biopsychosocial complexity. However, we can reflect on the latter in a way that is not reified, as a unique or 'unprecedented' condition. Lessons from previous pandemics are relevant to note. More common conditions arising from viral infections, which may not even reach the status of being an epidemic, let alone a pandemic, have provided us with clues about the topic.

What the pandemic has done is remind us of long-standing controversies, which include debates about the 'whys and wherefores' of mass vaccination programmes. These have been fraught with controversies about both commercial interests and the willingness of ordinary people to trust political elites.

The pandemic has also invited us to reflect on psychosocial phenomena that preceded it, especially in relation to living with long-term conditions.

That older research reminds us that the acute risk of death from infections is replaced in its survivors by a range of daily living challenges. Moreover, they are inflected by a range of inequalities determined by access to money, work and optimal healthcare. In addition other social factors are relevant: poor or well-off; being male or female; being gay or straight; and, more fundamentally living in a war zone rather than in conditions of peaceful stability.

References

Agénor, M., A.E. Pérez, J.W. Koma, J.A. Abrams, A.J. McGregor, and B.O. Ojikutu. 2019. "Sexual Orientation Identity, Race/Ethnicity, and Lifetime HIV Testing in a National Probability Sample of U.S. Women and Men: An Intersectional Approach." *LGBT Health* 6 (6): 306–318.

Allington, D., S. McAndrew, B. Duffy, B. et al. 2022. "Trust and Experiences of National Health Service Healthcare Do Not Fully Explain Demographic Disparities in Coronavirus Vaccination Uptake in the UK: A Cross-Sectional Study." *BMJ Open* 12 (3): e053827.

Bambra, C., V. Albani, and P. Franklin. 2021. "COVID-19 and the Gender Health Paradox." *Scandinavian Journal of Public Health* 49 (1): 17–26.

Boytchev, H. 2021. "Covid-19: Why the Balkans' Vaccine Rollout Lags behind Most of Europe." *BMJ* 375: n2412.

Bowleg, L. 2020. "We're Not All in This Together: On COVID-19, Intersectionality, and Structural Inequality." *American Journal of Public Health* 110 (7): 917.

Bray, I., A. Gibson, and J. White. 2020. "Coronavirus Disease 2019 Mortality: A Multivariate Ecological Analysis in Relation to Ethnicity, Population Density, Obesity, Deprivation and Pollution." *Public Health* 185: 261–263.

Bhui, K.S., S. Dinos, D. Ashby, J. Nazroo, S. Wessely, and P.D. White. 2011. "Chronic Fatigue Syndrome in an Ethnically Diverse Population: The Influence of Psychosocial Adversity and Physical Inactivity." *BMC Medicine* 9: 26.

Callaghan, T., A. Moghtaderi, J.A. Lueck, et al. 2021. "Correlates and Disparities of Intention to Vaccinate against COVID-19." *Social Science and Medicine* 272: 113638.

Dennis, A., C. Robin, L.F. Jones, and H. Carter. 2022. "Exploring Vaccine Hesitancy in Care Home Employees in North West England: A Qualitative Study." *BMJ Open* 12 (5): e055239.

Dey, T., and A. Sinha. 2020. "Ethnicity and COVID-19 - A Commentary on 'World Health Oganization Declares Global Emergency: A Review of the 2019 Novel Coronavirus (COVID-19)'." *International Journal of Surgery* 76: 71–76.

Dassieu, L., M.G. Pagé, A. Lacasse, et al. 2021. "Chronic Pain Experience and Health Inequities during the COVID-19 Pandemic in Canada: Qualitative Findings from the Chronic Pain & COVID-19 Pan-Canadian Study." *International Journal for Equity in Health* 20 (1): 147.

Elliott, J., L. Munford, S. Ahmed, A. Littlewood, and C. Todd. 2022. "The Impact of COVID-19 Lockdowns on Physical Activity amongst Older Adults: Evidence from Longitudinal Data in the UK." *BMC Public Health* 22 (1): 1802.

Fallon, N., C. Brown, H. Twiddy, E. Brian, B. Frank, T. Nurmikko, and A. Stancak. 2021. "Adverse Effects of COVID-19-Related Lockdown on Pain, Physical Activity and Psychological Well-Being in People with Chronic Pain." *British Journal of Pain* 15 (3): 357–368.

Farr, W. 1856 *Report on the Nomenclature and Statistical Classification of Diseases.* HMSO. Cited in Armstrong, D. (2021). The COVID-19 pandemic and cause of death. *Sociology of Health & Illness* 43 (7): 1614–1626.

Ferlatte, O., I. Handlovsky, D. Ridge, T. Chanady, R. Knight, and J.L. Oliffe. 2022. "Understanding Stigma and Suicidality among Gay Men Living with HIV: A Photovoice Project." *SSM - Qualitative Research in Health* 2: 2667–3215.

Glassman, L.W., and J.E. Szymczak. 2022. "The Influence of Social Class and Institutional Relationships on the Experiences of Vaccine-Hesitant Mothers: A Qualitative Study." *BMC Public Health* 22 (1): 2309.

Halkitis, P.N. 2019. *The AIDS Generation: Stories of Survival and Resilience.* Oxford: Oxford University Press.

Jason, L.A., M. Islam, K. Conroy, J. Cotler, C. Torres, M. Johnson, and B. Mabie. 2021. "COVID-19 Symptoms over Time: Comparing Long-Haulers to ME/CFS." *Fatigue: Biomedicine, Health and Behavior* 9 (2): 59–68.

Lockyer, B., S. Islam, A. Rahman, J. Dickerson, K. Pickett, T. Sheldon, ... L. Sheard. 2021. "Bradford Institute for Health Research Covid-19 Scientific Advisory Group. Understanding COVID-19 Misinformation and Vaccine Hesitancy in Context: Findings from a Qualitative Study Involving Citizens in Bradford, UK." *Health Expectations* 24 (4): 1158–1167.

Kennedy, A., A. Rogers, and M. Crossley. 2007. "Participation, Roles, and the Dynamics of Change in a Group-Delivered Self-Management Course for People Living with HIV." *Qualitative Health Research* 17 (6): 744–758.

Kovacs, B., N. Caplan, S. Grob, and M. King. 2021. "Social Networks and Loneliness during the COVID-19 Pandemic." *Socius: Sociological Research for a Dynamic World* 7. doi: 10.1177/2378023120985254.

Kingstone, T., A.K. Taylor, C.A. O'Donnell, et al. 2020. "Finding the 'Right' GP: A Qualitative Study of the Experiences of People with Long-COVID." *BJGP Open* 4.

Lewin, K. 1935 *A Dynamic Theory of Personality.* New York: McGraw-Hill.

Marmot, M.G., H. Bosma, H. Hemingway, E. Brunner, and S. Stansfeld. 1997. "Contribution of Job Control and Other Risk Factors to Social Variations in Coronary Heart Disease Incidence." *Lancet* 350 (9073): 235–239.

Mauvais-Jarvis, F., S.L. Klein, and E.R. Levin. 2020. "Estradiol, Progesterone, Immunomodulation, and COVID-19 Outcomes." *Endocrinology* 161 (9): 127.

Moalem, S. 2020. *The Better Half: On the Genetic Superiority of Women.* London: Penguin.

Nazroo, J., and L. Becares. 2020. "Evidence for Ethnic Inequalities in Mortality Related to COVID-19 Infections: Findings from an Ecological Analysis of England." *BMJ Open* 10 (12): e041750.

Patrick, R., M. Power, K. Garthwaite, J. Kaufman, G. Page, and K. Pybus. 2022. *A Year Like no Other: Life on a Low Income during COVID-19.* London: Policy Press.

Peters, S., A. Rogers, P. Salmon, L. Gask, C. Dowrick, M. Towey, ... R. Morriss. 2009. "What Do Patients Choose to Tell Their Doctors? Qualitative Analysis of Potential Barriers to Reattributing Medically Unexplained Symptoms." *Journal of General Internal Medicine* 24 (4): 443–449.

Rogers, A., and D. Pilgrim. 1995. "Immunisation and Its Discontents: An Examination of Dissent from the UK Mass Childhood Immunisation Programme." *Health Care Analysis* 3: 99–115. doi: 10.1007/BF02198210.

Rogers, A., and D. Pilgrim 2003 *Mental Health and Inequality*. Basingstoke: Palgrave/Macmillan.

Rudan, I. 2020. "A Cascade of Causes That Led to the COVID-19 Tragedy in Italy and in Other European Union Countries." *Journal of Global Health* 10 (1): 010335. doi: 10.7189/jogh.10.010335. PMID: 32257150. PMCID: PMC7125421.

Rozenfeld, Y., J. Beam, H. Maier, et al. 2020. "A Model of Disparities: Risk Factors Associated with COVID-19 Infection." *International Journal for Equity in Health* 19 (1): 126.

Shabnam, S., C. Razieh, H. Dambha-Miller, T. Yates, C. Gillies, Y.V. Chudasama, … E.J. Morris. 2022. *Socioeconomic Inequalities of Long COVID: Findings from a Population-Based Survey in the United Kingdom* (preprint).

Silva, J.K.B.D., J.M.D. Santos, W.C. Moreira, R.O.G. Romero, O.D.C.P. Leadebal, and J.A. Nogueira. 2022. "Multilevel Model in the Identification of Behavioral and Structural Risk Factors for HIV: Integrative Review." *Revista Brasileira de Enfermagem* 76 (1): e20210853.

Strong, P. 1990. "Epidemic Psychology: A Model." *Sociology of Health and Illness* 12 (3): 249–259.

Vaughan, L., D. Veruttipong, J.G. Shaw, et al. 2021. "Relationship of Socio-demographics, Comorbidities, Symptoms and Healthcare Access with Early COVID-19 Presentation and Disease Severity." *BMC Infectious Diseases* 21 (1): 40.

Wacquant, L. 2022 *The Invention of the 'Underclass'*. Cambridge: Polity Press.

Walker, S., H. Goodfellow, P. Pookarnjanamorakot, et al. 2023. "Impact of Fatigue as the Primary Determinant of Functional Limitations Among Patients with Post-covid-19 Syndrome: A Cross-Sectional Observational Study." *BMJ Open* 13: e069217. doi: 10.1136/bmjopen-2022-069217.

Index